100 Questions & Answers About Schizophrenia: Painful Minds

Lynn E. DeLisi

Professor of Psychia
New York Universit,
New York, NY
and
Associate Director of the Center for Advanced Brain Imaging
The Nathan S. Kline Institute for Psychiatric Research
Orangeburg, NY

*Dr. DeLisi is also co-founder and co-editor-in-chief of the journal, *Schizophrenia Research*, and co-founder and secretary of The Schizophrenia International Research Society.

JONES AND BARTLETT PUBLISHERS
Sudbury, Massachusetts
BOSTON   TORONTO   LONDON   SINGAPORE

World Headquarters

Jones and Bartlett
Publishers
40 Tall Pine Drive
Sudbury, MA 01776
978-443-5000
info@jbpub.com
www.jbpub.com

Jones and Bartlett
Publishers Canada
6339 Ormindale Road
Mississauga, ON L5V
1J2
CANADA

Jones and Bartlett
Publishers International
Barb House, Barb Mews
London W6 7PA
UK

Jones and Bartlett's books and products are available through most bookstores and online
booksellers. To contact Jones and Bartlett Publishers directly, call 800-832-0034, fax 978-443-
8000, or visit our website www.jbpub.com.

Substantial discounts on bulk quantities of Jones and Bartlett's publications are available to
corporations, professional associations, and other qualified organizations. For details and specific discount information, contact the special sales department at Jones and Bartlett via the
above contact information or send an email to specialsales@jbpub.com.

Production Credits
Executive Publisher: Christopher Davis
Associate Editor: Kathy Richardson
Associate Production Editor: Dan Stone
Associate Marketing Manager: Laura Kavigian
Manufacturing Buyer: Therese Connell
Composition: Appingo
Cover Design: Kate Ternullo
Cover Image: ©Photodisc; ©Ablestock; and ©Photos.com
Printing and Binding: Malloy, Inc.
Cover Printing: Malloy, Inc.

Library of Congress Cataloging-in-Publication Data
DeLisi, Lynn E.
    100 questions & answers about schizophrenia / Lynn E DeLisi.
       p. cm.
    Includes bibliographical references and index.
    ISBN-13: 978-0-7637-3654-5 (alk. paper)
    ISBN-10: 0-7637-3654-6 (alk. paper)
    1. Schizophrenia--Popular works. I. Title: 100 questions and answers about schizophrenia.
    II. Title: One hundred questions & answers about schizophrenia. III. Title.
    RC514.D45 2006
    616.89'8--dc22
                                    20060064806048
6048

Printed in the United States of America
09 08 07 06   10 9 8 7 6 5 4 3 2 1

Contents

Foreword
iv
Introduction
xiii
Dedication
xvii

Part 1: The Illness and Its Characteristics   *3*

1. What is schizophrenia?   4
2. Is schizophrenia a split personality?   6
3. What are the first signs of this illness? How do I know whether I (or my relative) have schizophrenia?   7
4. Is being "schizophreniform" the same as having "schizophrenia"?   10
5. What is schizoaffective disorder?   10
6. How is schizophrenia different from manic depression or Bipolar disease?   12
7. What is catatonia?   12
8. What is the course of the illness over time?   14
9. Is it possible to hear voices that are not there and not have schizophrenia?   16
10. How is excessive religiosity distinguished from schizophrenia?   17
11. What is meant by "positive" and "negative" symptoms?   18
12. Do people with schizophrenia have language problems?   18
13. Do people with schizophrenia get depression?   19
14. Are memory problems symptoms of schizophrenia?   20
15. Do people with schizophrenia have a low IQ?   21
16. Are muscular problems associated with schizophrenia?   21
17. Do people with schizophrenia have a reduced life span or die from their illness?   21
18. Are there medical conditions that look like schizophrenia?   22

19. Do people with schizophrenia have fewer offspring?   22

20. Are there some societies in which no individuals develop schizophrenia?   23

Part 2: Treatment: When, Where, by Whom, and with What?   25

21. What type of professional can treat the first symptoms of schizophrenia?   26

22. Does a psychiatrist always need to be seen and how frequently?   27

23. Why do some psychiatrists not treat people with schizophrenia?   28

24. What if I do not have insurance or my policy does not cover psychiatric care?   29

25. Do I have to be treated in a hospital if I have schizophrenia and if so, for how long?   29

26. What treatments were used before pharmaceutical companies introduced neuroleptic medication?   31

27. What about lobotomies?   32

28. What are the choices for medication?   33

29. What are the medication side effects?   35

30. What are the treatments for side effects?   36

31. Are there alternative treatments to medication?   36

32. What is cognitive behavioral therapy (CBT)?   36

33. Can a specific diet help?   38

34. What about vitamins and fish oil?   38

35. Can psychotherapy help?   40

36. Can family therapy help?   40

37. How long does medication have to be taken?   41

38. Is electroconvulsive therapy used for schizophrenia?   42

39. What are the pros and cons of participating in research studies?   43

Contents

Part 3: The Consideration of Nongenetic Risk Factors — 45

40. Do birth complications cause schizophrenia? — 46
41. Is schizophrenia more common in some cultural or racial groups than others? — 47
42. Can bad family relationships cause schizophrenia? — 48
43. What about immigration from another county? — 49
44. Is it better to live in a rural area? — 49
45. Is schizophrenia infectious? — 50
46. Do viruses cause schizophrenia? — 50

Part 4: The Genetic Risk — 53

47. What are the lessons from history? — 54
48. Who were the Genain quadruplets? — 55
49. Is schizophrenia inherited? And if so, how? — 57
50. If my aunt, uncle, or cousin has schizophrenia, what are the chances of my children getting it? — 58
51. If I have a brother with schizophrenia and my partner does too, what are the chances of our children getting schizophrenia? — 59
52. If I have an identical twin with schizophrenia, but I am well, what are my children's chances of having schizophrenia? — 60
53. How has biologic genetic research on schizophrenia been conducted in the past? — 60
54. What does linkage to a chromosome mean? — 61
55. What are microarrays? — 63
56. What are the candidate genes for schizophrenia? — 64
57. How is it assumed that these genes cause schizophrenia? — 66
58. What is an "intermediate phenotype" for schizophrenia? — 66
59. Will there be DNA testing for schizophrenia in the future? — 68
60. Will DNA testing be useful in determining which medication to administer? — 68
61. Can genetic research provide new treatments? — 69
62. What are ethical concerns in this new genome age for the future? — 69

Part 5: The Biology Underlying Schizophrenia: Current Research Findings   *71*

63. Are there any tests that can be taken from blood, urine, or spinal fluid?   72

64. Are there any differences in the brains of people that have schizophrenia?   72

65. Should an MRI scan be performed?   75

66. Are functional MRI scans useful?   75

67. Should an EEG be done on patients with schizophrenia?   76

68. Is schizophrenia a "chemical imbalance"?   76

69. When do these brain changes occur, and is schizophrenia considered a progressive brain disorder?   78

70. What is the neurodevelopmental hypothesis about schizophrenia?   79

Part 6: Substance Abuse and Schizophrenia   *81*

71. Can drug use in adolescence cause schizophrenia?   82

72. Can someone who has schizophrenia smoke marijuana?   83

73. Are there any specific drugs that more frequently cause schizophrenia-like symptoms?   83

74. Is it okay to drink alcohol if you have schizophrenia?   84

75. Why do people with schizophrenia smoke cigarettes excessively?   84

Part 7: Violence and Aggression in Schizophrenia   *87*

76. Do people with schizophrenia frequently commit violent acts?   88

77. Is there research on how violent behavior can be predicted?   89

78. Do people with schizophrenia more frequently commit crimes?   91

79. What should I do if my relative or friend is behaving violently?   91

Part 8: Suicidal Behavior and Schizophrenia   *93*

80. What are the signs of suicidal thoughts in schizophrenia?   94

81. What can be done to prevent suicide attempts?   95

Part 9: Issues for Women 97

82. Is schizophrenia different in women? 98

83. Should patients who are pregnant take medication for schizophrenia? 99

84. What is the risk of a postpartum relapse? 100

85. What about breast-feeding? 101

86. Does the concept "schizophrenogenic mother" exist? 102

87. Can estrogens for birth control help suppress symptoms? 102

Part 10: The Homeless and Schizophrenia 103

88. How prevalent is schizophrenia among the homeless? 104

89. What causes homelessness? 106

90. Can homeless people be forced into shelters and hospitals? 106

Part 11: Living with Schizophrenia 109

91. What are the origins of the stigma attached to having schizophrenia? 110

92. Can a person with schizophrenia be professionally creative? 111

93. Should I adopt a baby whose parent had schizophrenia? 111

94. Should a person with schizophrenia drive a car? 112

Part 12: Ethical Issues 113

95. What does "involuntary" hospital commitment involve? 114

96. What is the legal insanity defense? 115

97. Have there been abuses of the insanity defense? 116

98. Do patients with schizophrenia have the capacity to give written informed consent for research and other procedures? 119

99. Can genetic information be abused? 120

100. Are there support groups, books, and websites to help? 121

Resources 123

Glossary 129

Index 137

After hours of waiting, my husband and I scanned the passengers spilling out from the late-night flight returning from Costa Rica. Our son, Charles, had flown there for a surfing vacation with friends, but a few days into the trip we received a frightening call. Charles' friend David (his name has been changed to protect privacy) phoned to say that Charles was acting strangely—sleeping on the beach in the rain, chain smoking but refusing to eat, and repeatedly saying that he just needed to go home. David said that he had taken Charles to the airport but because of security restrictions did not know whether Charles actually got on the plane. Now we were waiting in Kennedy Airport, wondering whether Charles would be walking off the plane or wandering around an airport in a foreign country, in need of medical attention, while we sat in New York with no passports to even fly there to help him.

Years of wondering whether something was medically wrong with Charles were coming to a head. Although the comments began around the age of 10 years, with teachers noticing his dreaminess and inability to concentrate, they escalated in junior high to observations that he often put his head on his desk during class and seemed like he might be depressed. Those problems continued in high school. Unlike most teens, Charles seemed to enjoy discussing his unusual ideas about philosophy, religion, and government. Still, he had many friends, saved for and bought a car, and expressed his artistic impulse in photography, sketching, poetry, and playing the guitar. Was his lack of engagement at school a facet of his personality, teenage moodiness, or a symptom of mental illness? Even counselors had trouble sorting that out, and when he managed to graduate high school, we thought that perhaps the worst was behind us. A lack of focus, however, continued to plague him, and the questions persisted. What was wrong with our son?

Why did he claim to have special gifts, like the ability to read minds? Did he need treatment or just patience while he grew into a less impulsive, sharper-focused young man?

At last, Charles appeared in the line of passengers, looking distracted and thin, but seemingly coherent enough to speak right away of getting a new job, car insurance, and other things that were true. On the way home, I offered to let him sit in the front seat of the car, not knowing our moment of truth was about to unfold. He began to tell of how beautiful Costa Rica was and how he really had not wanted to leave. Then he turned around to face me and spoke the words that ended our years of wondering. "I had to leave," he said, looking very worried, "because David was trying to kill me." Thus, this was it—no more kidding ourselves. He was so out of touch with reality that he thought his good friend wanted to kill him. I sank into the darkness of the back seat, grateful that he could not see the wave of despair washing over me.

The next day, after articulately telling his story to doctors and counselors at the hospital, Charles reluctantly admitted himself. The symptoms now had a name—schizophrenia. While he went for admission testing, I opened the booklet a staff member had given me. "Schizophrenia is a chronic, severe, and disabling brain disease," it began. I wanted to throw up, scream, simply push away this dark news with all my might, but I just sat with an unstoppable flow of tears streaming down my face. Leaving your child behind in a locked mental ward breaks something inside of you. My husband's dam burst as soon as we got to the car. He sobbed and moaned, and we held shaky hands, reassuring each other that we were doing the best possible thing for Charles. Why did the best possible thing feel so horrible?

Charles stayed a week, but his odyssey toward acceptance of both the diagnosis and the medicine required to treat it took much longer. He downplayed his earlier "crazy" statements and said that he was just being stupid. He did not need medicine because it made him feel weird. Like most people, he did not want the label of a disease applied to him. The lack of treatment and failure to keep even his counseling appointments, however, let the disease draw him into a frightening place where he thought people could read his mind, the television spoke directly to him, and insistent, negative voices said that he should go to hell or kill himself. After hitting the bottom and enduring another two-week hospitalization, Charles accepted that he needed the help of medication, a counselor, and all the support that his family and friends could offer.

Still, this new path, so filled with scary, unexpected turns left us filled with anxiety about his future. Would he end up a homeless wanderer someday, impossible to locate or help? I worked in a library where the mentally ill sometimes had to be confronted when their behavior affected other patrons. Would my son become someone whose appearance and behavior scared others in public places? Was there a possibility that his psychosis was a one-time occurrence and that he would someday be "normal"? Would my other children develop this disease?

A diagnosis of an unfamiliar disease leaves patients and their loved ones filled with questions and fears like mine. This makes a book such as *100 Questions & Answers About Schizophrenia* very important. As a librarian, I practice the adage "information is power," and Dr. DeLisi's book fills the need for comprehending a misunderstood illness such as schizophrenia. Using this book as a resource will empower you with the knowledge that is necessary to cope with the diagnosis of mental illness.

Sadly, Charles chose to end his battle with the persistent voices and overwhelming depression. On the surface, he had seemed to be improving. He reported hearing fewer voices and asked to have his amount of antipsychotic medication lowered; he even signed up to begin classes at a local college and started a new job. One day, however, we came home from work and found his lifeless body in the backyard. His girlfriend said the night before he had told her, "I'm in so much pain my heart hurts." The psychic pain of mental illness can be as hard to bear as the physical pain of a cancer or back injury.

I share his story not as a warning but as a testament to the devastation that mental illness can cause. A bright, creative, energetic boy spent his final teen years seeking refuge in sleep and music. For you or your loved one, I hope for a positive outcome made possible by continuing research such as that done by Dr. DeLisi and her colleagues. May hope for a better future buoy you as you continue the journey of acceptance, treatment, and attainment of a fulfilling life.

Eileen Trupia

Mother of Charles Wesley Trupia, 3/24/83–7/31/03

Too often patients are lost to treatment in the current U.S. mental healthcare system that is governed by insurance policies and overworked caregivers. Adequate intensive follow-up care is sometimes not given to those who clearly need it, and thus, the patients slip by with warning signs unnoticed. We continue to work toward parity for mental illness in the healthcare system and to improve the quality of care so that no family needlessly suffers as was in this case.

Lynn E. DeLisi, MD

Several years ago I knew that I would somehow do something to let the public know about what I considered to be the true facts about schizophrenia when my daughter came home from high school saying that her health class teacher described schizophrenia as a "split personality." This statement could not be farther from the truth. Schizophrenia is not a Jekyll and Hyde type of condition; however, when Bleuler coined this term in 1911, he erroneously used the Latin for "split mind." What he meant was that there was a "split"—or inconsistency between the affect and emotions, thought and speech, and perhaps perception and reality.

This term has continued over the years to describe a psychiatric disorder that is very heterogeneous in its expression, clinical course, and biology. It has also had an unusual course in history. During the turn of the 20th century, patients with these symptoms were shunned by society and isolated in large, gated multibuilding complexes called psychiatric hospitals or institutions, often being committed by relatives and staying for years. During World War II, the Nazi extermination policy began with a focus on patients in psychiatric hospitals, as they were deemed unfit to live and take up national resources. Many psychiatrists even played terrible roles in facilitating these policies because of their lack of understanding of the biology and inheritance of this disorder.

It was only in the late 1960s when neuroleptic medications were accepted as the treatment of choice, and marked improvement in behavior could be seen, that patients were rehabilitated back into the community. Slowly the public institutions were emptied, and residences sprung up within towns for patients who were stabilized and were treatable on an outpatient basis. Periodically questions about the nature of this illness resurface when someone with schizophrenia is in the news for having committed a violent act toward an innocent bystander; then the prudence of releasing some patients prematurely from long-term hospital commitment is questioned. One such famous case was John Hinckley Jr., a young man who shot former President Reagan and one of his cabinet members (James Brady), who was permanently disabled subsequent to this attack. Of course, many more people who do not have a diagnosis of schizophrenia commit violent acts than those with the diagnosis, but, nevertheless, unpredictable behavior is a frightening hallmark of unstabilized or undertreated symptoms of schizophrenia, particularly of the paranoid type.

These types of behaviors, plus the bizarreness and inappropriateness of some of the symptoms, lead to a very difficult social situation that not only affects the decision to seek an appropriate treatment, but also impacts how someone with this diagnosis is viewed by people with whom he or she interacts socially, professionally, and legally. These characteristics lead to the stigma that has been formed about schizophrenia over the years. Unfortunately, physicians, because of this stigma, will often delay making such a diagnosis and will then likely cause more damage by initially assuring parents that their son or daughter will "grow out of it." They will instead label the emotional difficulties as an "adjustment reaction," which requires no medication but simply observation and psychotherapy over time. The harm is that we now know that it is likely that early pharmacologic treatment may prevent the severe chronic debilitating form of this illness. The discrimination caused by stigmatizing this illness extends into further aspects of life. Insurance companies do not treat schizophrenia as a medical illness that needs treatment in the same way as pneumonia or other ailments that originate below the head. Employers would likely eliminate anyone who wrote on a job application that he or she was in the past, or is now currently, diagnosed with schizophrenia. Families keep secret that one of their relatives is afflicted because the stigma may contribute to a potential mate's questioning marrying into such a family. As with a history of depression, having had schizophrenia in one's past is used against those rare individuals who recover, so that they are unlikely to ever hold a government office or to succeed in ways that they could have if they not been diagnosed.

Nevertheless, many famous and creative figures are said to have schizophrenia or at least a psychotic illness that at times was certainly indistinguishable from schizophrenia. Among them are musicians (such as Brian Wilson from The Beach Boys), artists (Van Gogh), Nobel Prize winners (John Nash), kings (Christian 7 of Denmark in the late 1700s), and historical figures such as Joan of Arc. They contrast at an extreme with those with violent pasts such as the Unabomber or the Yorkshire Ripper. Famous movies have depicted people with schizophrenia for decades, from the early horrors in *The Snake Pit* to *One Flew Over the Cuckoo's Nest* to *I Never Promised You a Rose Garden* and most recently, *A Beautiful Mind.* Although some people aid in quelling the stigma surrounding this illness, others point fingers at people with schizophrenia as peculiar and use the words *cuckoo, nuts,* or *loco* to describe their thoughts and behavior.

Most people who do stigmatize people with schizophrenia know little about the scientific basis for this illness and whether their actions make practical sense. This book is designed to refute the basis for the stigma that exists in all aspects of life and to provide the public with a glimpse of what it is like to have schizophrenia, what causes it, how it can be treated, and how to live a productive life when you or a family member has schizophrenia (Aschaffenburg G 1911-1928).

Lynn E. DeLisi, MD
March, 2006

Dedication

This volume is dedicated to all the families worldwide who suffer because they have one or more family members with schizophrenia, and to those individuals whose lives have been destroyed by this illness.

Part One

The Illness and Its Characteristics

"By New Year's Day . . . Nash's behavior had become more and more peculiar. He was irritable and hypersensitive one minute, eerily withdrawn the next. He complained that he knew that something was going on and that he was being bugged. Also, he was staying up nights writing strange letters to the United Nations. One night he had painted black spots all over their bedroom wall,"

as the wife of John Nash, Nobel Laureate 1994, told to Sylvia Nasar (1998) in an interview

1. What is schizophrenia?

Schizophrenia

any of a group of psychotic disorders usually characterized by withdrawal from reality, illogical patterns of thinking, delusions, and hallucinations, and accompanied in varying degrees by other emotional, behavioral, or intellectual disturbances.

DSM-IV

the diagnostic and statistical manual developed by leading clinical psychiatrists in the United States for the systematic evaluation of psychiatric patients and assigning diagnoses to groups of symptoms.

Delusion

a false belief based on faulty judgment about one's environment.

Hallucinations

experiencing something from any of the five senses that is not occurring in reality.

Prodrome

an early or premonitory symptom of a disease.

Residual

having some nonspecific symptoms (usually negative symptoms), but no longer active psychotic ones.

The American Psychiatric Association defines **schizophrenia** as a disorder with active symptoms for at least one month, consisting of **delusions**, **hallucinations**, disorganized speech, grossly disorganized/bizarre behavior, and/or a lack of organized speech, activity, or emotions (**DSM-IV**). Usually at least two of these sets of symptoms are present. The illness, with a **prodromal** stage and a **residual** stage after treatment, both having some often nonspecific behavioral symptoms, lasts at least six months with continuous signs of some disturbance. During this period an individual with schizophrenia is clearly considered impaired in his or her ability to perform at work, attend school, or participate in social activities in a productive way.

The hallucinations of schizophrenia are most often auditory, although visual, olfactory, and tactile hallucinations have been described as well. The latter, however, are more often due to substance abuse (alcohol or street drugs) than schizophrenia when they predominate. The auditory hallucinations that distinguish schizophrenia are not just sounds. They are words spoken aloud as if someone else is actually speaking them, although no one is there. They can be one person that is or is not recognized by the individual, and that person is commenting in some way on the hearer's behavior. They also can be multiple voices talking about the hearer, usually in a frightening or derogatory manner. Sometimes the hallucinations have been occurring for years before any other symptoms and unrecognized by the individual as anything that is abnormal or not happening to everyone. Many times, when severe, they intrude into the person's life and daily activities. The patient can be found actually responding to the voices as if in conversation. Without experience, any examiner might have difficulty imagining what hallucinations are like.

The word *delusion* is certainly common, but the delusions of schizophrenia can sometimes be characteristic. Many are bizarre to the normal person. For example, feeling that some unknown force is controlling one's actions or emotions or seeing objects in the environment with new meaning are frequently mentioned. Similarly, one could be watching television or a movie and feeling that the people on the screen are giving the watcher some special messages. Common environmental situations, such as water dripping from a faucet, take on a new magical meaning. The feeling that parts of one's body are not one's own are described, as well as feeling like an actor on the "stage of life" and not being "real." Other common symptoms are the patient's ability to mind read or feeling that other people know the patient's own thoughts, as if they are spoken on a loudspeaker. Patients with schizophrenia are suspicious that people are harming them (e.g., by food poisoning) or that a complicated plot by the government against the individual is occurring. These latter **paranoid** delusions may be accompanied by delusions of grandeur (thinking that one is or can have extraordinary powers or abilities that are in reality not possessed) and hyperreligiosity—of knowing that God has singled one out for a special mission. I once had a patient who knew he would "be president of the United States" because "God had told him." This was, however, someone who had been barely an average student throughout school and thought that London, England, was in the midwestern United States!

Paranoid

excessive or irrational suspicion or distrust of others.

Most psychiatrists today would agree that schizophrenia is defined by at least three separate sets of symptoms: (1) positive ones that include hallucinations and delusions; (2) negative ones that include a general appearance of being flat (without much emotion), called "flat affect," withdrawal, a lack of much speech, at least speech that says anything, and slowness of movements and the appearance of slowness to thinking; and (3) a set of symptoms related to general disorganization (i.e., speech that is mixed or not getting to the point and behavioral disorganization). The latter is now considered a third cluster, defined as a **disorganizational syndrome**.

Disorginazational syndrome

a set of symptoms related to general disorganization (speech and/or behaviorial disorginization).

Subtypes of schizophrenia and different types of related diagnoses exist as well. The paranoid subtype is more heavily delusions and hallucinations, rather than any disorganization, and the symptoms are often paranoid in nature, but not always. The disorganized subtype has most prominently the disorganization symptoms already mentioned. The catatonic subtype focuses on predominantly motor and speech changes that are either excessive or too little. The undifferentiated subtype is generally a mixture of the others, with one type not being more prominent. Finally, the residual subtype is one in which the patient has become stabilized and no longer has the delusions and hallucinations but still does not seem normal and has many so-called **negative symptoms** (appearing withdrawn, speaking minimally, lacking initiative, etc.) that have not resolved.

Negative symptoms
those characteristics of psychiatric illness that present as withdrawn behavior, an expressionless face, a lack of initiative, a lack of interest, slow speech, and not saying much when talking, slowed thoughts, and slowed movements. Sometimes these symptoms are confused with either depression or side effects of medication.

2. Is schizophrenia a split personality?

The word *schizophrenia* is clearly a misnomer. Eugene Bleuler, who coined this term back in the early part of the 20th century, did so because he saw an abnormal "split" between the outward affect of the patient and his or her emotions and a split between thought, speech, and affect. The split is actually due to an underlying misconnection of brain functional activity. A split personality is quite a rare syndrome whereby a person assumes different identities; an environmental trigger initiates this switch. Usually these identities have been manifest in the mind of such an individual because of traumatic events, such as sexual abuse, having taken place in his or her childhood that have been extremely stressful to acknowledge. These individuals may benefit from intense psychotherapy over the years but are in no way similar clinically or biologically to people with schizophrenia.

3. What are the first signs of this illness? How do I know whether I (or my relative) have schizophrenia?

The following case illustrates the essence of this question: Maryanne was a first-year medical student who received an educational loan that covered only the subsidized housing development in which she was forced to live. She took a job as a waitress in a nearby bar on hours when she was not on student patient call in the evening. She gained support from a group of same-sex classmates and would often study with them in afternoons after class or during lunch breaks. Tension was high during exams, and classmate support was often emotionally helpful. Occasionally marijuana was passed from student to student during mass cramming sessions. Laurie, a fellow classmate, noticed at some point that Maryanne was occasionally, and then more frequently, missing classes. Finally, she and three other friends made the trip across town to Maryanne's apartment. The lights were dim, and at first their knocks went unheard. Chanting was overheard by the girls, however, and thus they persisted. Eventually, Maryanne came to the door inappropriately dressed in Muslim robes. Candles glowed in a circle surrounding her living room, and food and other items were scattered across the floor. Maryanne explained that she had taken up meditating and had converted to a Muslim sect, reciting some verses from the Koran. She assured her friends that she was fine but preferred to stay home that day. Eventually, when school administrators noticed her absence, she was called in and required to attend psychotherapy in order to return to school. Instead, she dropped out of school and disappeared. Eventually, she was unemployed and lost her apartment, became homeless for a time, and received a small note in the local paper when she finally committed suicide by attempting a bizarre baptism in the ocean.

Stories such as Maryanne's are too common. Although they luckily do not all lead to suicide, many do lead to a cessation of normal life and a loss of the potential as a young adult their future held. Often relatives and close friends are unaware of why the individual is wary of confiding in anyone and remains seclusive or hard to find. The person who is developing schizophrenia rarely has any insight that he or she is ill and thus does not admit to anyone about the stressful thoughts and perceptions occurring, despite their disturbing nature. Those who are close—friends and relatives—may notice a change in behavior and emotional responses; however, they do not know that the affected person is having hallucinations and delusionary thoughts unless the person says things that sound bizarre or that clearly cannot be true. Often, particularly when of a paranoid nature, these things are kept to one's self.

Families, if intact, after recognizing problems will rally to the support of the ill individual but are soon depleted of funds and frustrated by the lack of community and legal support to aid their relative. Parents eventually become resigned to care for these children permanently, but as they age they worry about who will care for the child after they are gone.

Psychiatric researchers continuously debate on how best to predict that a schizophrenic-like illness is likely to occur. It would be important to find clear predictors that can distinguish the symptoms of illness from the variation in functioning and the "ups and downs" of stages of life experiences, particularly in adolescence. None, however, has clearly been found.

The key probably has to do with change from one's usual functioning (i.e., withdrawal from friendships, peculiar statements that are not true, and a change in organization of behavior and speech). Work and school activities change for the worse, and an overall troubled withdrawal of the individual becomes apparent to those with whom he or she interacts. This individual may be heard talking to himself or herself or making untrue or bizarre statements about other people or events. These symptoms often accelerate to the point in which the individual can behave in an inappropriate or harmful manner (such as undressing in public or walking down the middle of a highway). In other instances, the individual will perform impulsive and aggressive acts without understanding the consequence of such actions. At this point the police are called, and the individual is brought to either jail or a psychiatric emergency room. Obviously, it is beneficial if early signs can be recognized and treated before they accelerate to a dangerous situation.

In general, schizophrenia develops gradually, on average over about a two-year period in an adolescent or young adult. Behavioral changes—such as withdrawing socially, a noticeable decline in academic performance, irritability, or what appears as **depression**—are first noticed by close friends or family. The individuals may also be found sleeping either too much or too little and are periodically agitated. These things might eventually lead a parent to consult a family physician about his or her child. The parent might be told that adolescent turmoil or adjustment problems are the cause. Most physicians delay making a diagnosis of schizophrenia, particularly if the patients does not admit to clear auditory hallucinations and bizarre delusions. The message to a parent may simply be that "he or she will grow out of it." Frequent follow-up, however, should be instituted in these cases. The patient may eventually admit to clear symptoms, which gives the opportunity for early treatment and possible prevention of the severe chronic form of the illness.

The typical case, however, is a young person who has done something clearly bizarre and either harmful to himself or herself or others to the point where the police or a psychiatric crisis unit is called for help. In at least half of the cases in several countries, some kind

Depression

a major psychiatric condition characterized by profound sadness all day. It is usually accompanied by physical symptoms, such as loss of appetite, loss of sleep, and slowness in movements and speech. If the condition continues as long as one week without relief and interferes with a person's ability to function, it is then called major depression.

of street drug use may be acutely responsible or at least contribute to the bizarre and harmful behavior. Many first-episode patients, after being treated and having the symptoms resolve, conclude that drug use was the cause and that they will be okay as long as they abstain from drugs (see Part Six for a more detailed discussion of drug abuse). This assumption, however, is in many cases false. The drugs may have initiated the disease that might have eventually occurred regardless at a later time under some other stress. The danger is that the patient will assume that he or she does not need the **neuroleptic** medication prescribed as long as street drugs are not taken again. The medications and treatment given during the acute episode are terminated, and the patient eventually comes back to the hospital in a more serious relapse of symptoms that are generally more difficult to suppress with medication. The patient who terminates his or her first treatment without being integrated into the chronic care system is most likely to commit suicide.

4. Is being "schizophreniform" the same as having "schizophrenia"?

In **schizophreniform** disorder, a patient has all the symptoms of schizophrenia, but the symptoms resolve in less than a month without residual symptoms. Generally, this person was functioning very well and very acutely developed symptoms that also resolved relatively quickly with or without medication.

5. What is schizoaffective disorder?

Schizoaffective disorder is a related diagnosis and may be the same disorder in its biologic origins. Such a patient has all the symptoms of schizophrenia but also has significantly overlapping symptoms of depression, **manic behavior**, or both. Depression is generally defined as feeling very sad emotionally, perhaps to the point of having suicidal ideas or actions, with loss of weight and sleep often as a result. Manic behavior, on

---

Neuroleptic

any medication that when given to animals will cause catalepsy. This name then was used to label all drugs that had an effect on reducing the symptoms of schizophrenia. They are sometimes known as the "major tranquilizers."

Schizophreniform

having the symptoms of schizophrenia, but too early in the course of illness to tell whether the symptoms are of a schizophrenia illness.

Schizoaffective

having both prominent symptoms of schizophrenia and depression and/or mania that overlap with the schizophrenia-like symptoms. However, they do not always coincide, so that sometimes the patients have only schizophrenia-like symptoms and at other times, although less so, only mania or depressive symptoms.

Manic behavior

feeling excessively elated and cheery with very fast speech and thoughts.

the other hand, is feeling excessively elated and cheery with very fast speech and thoughts, perhaps also doing some bizarre and risky acts during this period as well. Agitated behavior is sometimes seen with manic behavior. Grandiose delusions are also part of this syndrome.

Interestingly, psychiatrists generally differ in whether they would diagnose someone with schizophrenia or schizoaffective disorder, as well as any of the subtypes of schizophrenia, and over the course of illness these diagnoses in one individual seem to change. Similarly, they differ in whether someone with schizoaffective disorder should at some times be diagnosed with **bipolar affective disorder**. Thus, patients who are sometimes diagnosed with schizoaffective disorder may not only by some psychiatrist be seen as schizophrenic but may by others be seen as having manic-depressive disorder. One view is that a biologic continuum likely exists between all these diagnoses. The extremes and more classical cases of each are more consistently diagnosable among psychiatrists, but the vast majority fall into the middle somewhere. They can either be called schizophrenia-spectrum disorder or moreover be classified and treated by the symptoms that occur, rather than the category of diagnosis. It may be that the underlying biology of what appear to be different illnesses may really be the same but clinically be expressed differently in different individuals from a very disorganized schizophrenia-like degenerative illness to a cyclic episode of **psychotic** symptoms with normality in between, the so-called "unitary psychosis" (Crow, 1990). When we can clearly designate biological underpinnings for each syndrome of symptoms or a common biology to all, we anticipate that entirely different diagnostic categories may be developed that reflect the biology more directly.

Bipolar affective disorder

a psychiatric condition characterized by mood swings that occur episodically. Sometimes, particularly when very "high" (manic), people with bipolar disorder can have many of the characteristic positive symptoms of schizophrenia.

Psychotic

people are considered psychotic if they have lost touch with reality, have delusions (i.e., false beliefs), and hallucinations. They often are exhibiting bizarre and risky behavior and do not seem to be aware that they are doing anything unusual.

6. How is schizophrenia different from manic depression or bipolar disease?

Although, as mentioned above, some psychiatrists believe that a biological continuum exists between the extremes of these two disorders, there are differences. Many people with bipolar disorder can lead a normal, productive, and very creative life after their mood is stabilized. After an episode, providing that medication is continued, they appear to be able not to lose their original potential for functioning. Cognitive abilities are not impaired, as they are more often in schizophrenia. It is the severe cases of bipolar disorder with several frequent hospitalizations that eventually are indistinguishable from schizophrenia. Thus, the outcome is what is different, although some of the biology may be similar. Schizophrenia is more often thought of as a **neurodevelopmental** disorder with a poorer **premorbid** adjustment socially and academically in childhood. Prebipolar individuals are indistinguishable from others in those earlier years.

Much biologic research comparing the biology of these two disorders needs to be performed.

Although many of the brain structural changes present in schizophrenia have been found in bipolar disorder, severe bipolar disorder with psychotic features (such as hallucinations and delusions) appears to show these changes. Some of these differences and similarities are detailed in a book published by Maneros and Angst (2000), two researchers who have focused over the years on these issues.

7. What is catatonia?

Catatonic behavior is the extreme of being disorganized and can either be complete immobility and muteness or, at the opposite end, extreme disorganized excitability—an extreme frenzy-like behavior. **Catatonia** in its full-blown syndrome is actually rare today in

Neurodevelopmental

happening during the growth and formation of different structures of the brain.

Premorbid

the time period before any symptoms of a disorder, including subtle signs, have developed.

Catatonic behavior

behavior characterized by muscular tightness or rigidity and lack of response to the environment.

Catatonia

a condition that is characterized by extremes in behavior, of which the individual appears to be unaware. These behaviors include being mute or in a stupor and immobile to, at the other extreme, being in an excitatory state of an extreme frenzy or agitated excitement.

the United States and Western nations, although it can be seen more frequently in impoverished countries where patients do not get ample care and the newest pharmaceutical treatments available. Patients with catatonia are often quite remarkable in their appearance. They have what has been termed "waxy flexibility." That is, they stand in one position with their limbs stationary until a person moves them to another position, where they will stay until again moved by another person. A currently practicing U.S. psychiatrist may never have seen such cases. Nevertheless, one patient I remember clearly from the mid 1980s (when catatonia was already rare) was a young man who had driven himself to the outpatient clinic. After approaching the check-in desk, however, the receptionist looked up to find him immobile, stiff, and mute. I led him to a private room. He responded several minutes later, but only after having been administered a **tranquilizer** intramuscularly. He denied that anything unusual was happening and was aware that we were discussing him, but he had no explanation for why he had not responded. He then drove home without incident, but frequently entered my office again in that same manner.

I also recall a memorable experience when visiting the National Psychiatric Hospital in El Salvador in early 2002. Touring this hospital that was so ill equipped compared with U.S. public psychiatric hospitals was a startling awakening to the reality of the status of current psychiatric care in impoverished developing countries. High doses of old medicines were used, as psychiatrists did not know that newer drugs existed. The floors of the wards had drains to collect the urine that often was uncontrollably produced. What mainly stood out, however, were the several immobile individuals with classical catatonic schizophrenia. Unfortunately, we do not understand the biological mechanism that underlies this condition, and because it has become so rare over recent years, it is understudied.

Tranquilizer

any drug that is used to calm or pacify an anxious and/or agitated person. There are minor and major classes of tranquilizers that have different chemical properties and are indicated for different psychiatric conditions, the minor ones for anxiety in a person who has not lost a sense of reality but who needs calming. Major tranquilizers are the class of drugs used for psychotic symptoms.

8. What is the course of the illness over time?

No clear predictors of illness course exist, and hopefully, in the future, more biological variables will be affirmed. Females tend to have a milder course of illness and a later age of onset than males by about a mean of two years. Early age of onset and poor premorbid social and academic functioning are hallmarks of a more severe course of illness.

The old adage, however, is that one third of first-episode cases of schizophrenia go on to a chronic deteriorating course. One third are in the middle with illness but can function (albeit at a lower level than previously), and one third never have another episode again. The latter statistic is now thought to be overly optimistic. Although many individuals do quite well, particularly if they are treated early and have good family support, continual medication is the key. It is now believed that no more than 10 percent of individuals who have a clear first episode of schizophrenia can consider themselves recovered afterward without medication. Many additional people may find that they essentially have no symptoms while on medication. Unfortunately, they then think that they do not need it, stop the medication, and eventually relapse. Additionally, the time to a second episode varies. Often it does not occur immediately but may take a few years to again develop. Currently, with the advent of new medications that have almost no side effects, a stable dose can be achieved for a period of several years without the patient feeling the uncomfortable side effects of the old medications.

The course of illness may have changed and become milder as a result of early vigorous treatment with new medications and better compliance among patients. If left untreated, the natural course of schizophrenia is a lifetime of symptoms and deterioration.

Before the widespread use of neuroleptic medications, patients were hospitalized for years and lived the rest of their lives on the "back wards" of public hospitals, deteriorating in manner and **cognition**. It was hard to distinguish between this course of illness and the environmentally deprived effects of institutionalization. When government legislation for the establishment of community mental health centers became in vogue in the 1960s to 1970s, medicated patients were discharged from hospitals and returned to the community. The effects of long-term institutionalization were recognized, but not solved. Often the living environments that patients were transferred to were in many ways impoverished and unsupportive to the needs of these individuals. As a consequence of this dreary and problematic environment and partially the underlying illness itself, many patients returned frequently to the hospitals, and the so-called revolving door phenomenon began to take effect. Throughout their lifetime, patients began to have records filled with numerous admissions and discharges. State-allotted funds for the inpatient institutions have dwindled each year, resulting in the maximum number of beds per state hospital only a few hundred or even none in those that have closed. It is common to drive now through the grounds of the state facilities—once lively, self-sustaining communities in themselves—and see many buildings boarded up and vacant and weeds growing widely on the surrounding once patient-manicured grounds.

Currently, mental health care is in a crisis in the United States, as well as internationally. Schizophrenia is a lifetime disorder that can be effectively treated and cared for, but legislation needs to be in place that is sensitive to the needs of these disabled individuals instead of ignoring their need for care and stigmatizing them as a result. Nevertheless, the history of care for the mentally ill in the USA and other westernized countries outlined above hopefully is part of the past. There is current optimism that if continually med-

Cognition

the quality of the mind that allows animals to think, reason, and manipulate their environment to survive. Cognition can be measured by psychological tests. Of course, the tests are much simpler for nonhuman animals and are most complicated for humans. The well-known IQ is one measure of human cognition.

icated, people with schizophrenia now can lead normal productive lives and don't have to be burdened by uncomfortable symptoms or medication side effects.

9. Is it possible to hear voices that are not there and not have schizophrenia?

Recently, reports of surveys of the general non–treatment-seeking population conclude that auditory hallucinations and various forms of delusions are common. In fact, these investigators report that psychotic experiences are present in anywhere from 5 to 20 percent of the general population. This statement needs to be interpreted with caution, however, because sufficient follow-up has not been done of the people reporting these experiences to know whether eventually they will be diagnosed with full-blown schizophrenia or another serious psychiatric disturbance.

Many psychiatrists who treat patients with schizophrenia, if they question the patients specifically, find that patients frequently admit to having heard voices as far back as they can remember in childhood and never thought to mention these experiences, as they were perceived as "normal."

Having auditory hallucinations alone certainly does not mean that you have or will get schizophrenia. Many people never have any medical or psychiatric problems relating to the voices heard but have them particularly related to falling to sleep or just waking (not being fully alert). Another difference has to do with the nature of the voices. Someone calling your name or hearing sounds but not using complex language is less serious.

Command hallucinations

imaginary voices that tell the hearer what to do.

The hallmarks of classical schizophrenia are hearing more than one voice conversing with each other about the hearer and/or at least one voice commenting on the hearer's actions. There are also "**command hallucinations**," giving the hearer orders to carry out some action. These latter experiences are certainly more disturbing and characteristic of illness. They rarely, however, stand alone and are accompanied by either some form of bizarre behavior or multiple delusions.

10. How is excessive religiosity distinguished from schizophrenia?

Many times it is difficult to distinguish "real" delusions from cultural norms or outside stresses that are happening to individuals. For example, as a young psychiatrist, I worked not far from a revival church in which congregations would assemble and sing to a point where loudness progressed and members were drawn into chanting trances, almost as if they had no control over their actions and were so overcome by the event that one could perceive that they were all in acute psychotic states. When the music stopped and the meeting was over, however, each individual returned to an unnoticeable state.

When religion interferes with one's social life and occupational and educational achievements, you can call the beliefs a "symptom" of a disorder. Certainly this is one illustration that psychopathology is likely to be on a continuum in many ways between what is considered normal by society and what is considered abnormal by psychiatrists. Debates exist about whether schizophrenia actually exists other than in the imagination of psychiatrists. Although this view is certainly extreme, the cultural environment of a newly presenting patient needs to be considered before a diagnosis is made. The disorder that is described in this book is more than extreme views that can be related to culture. It affects individuals from all cultural backgrounds and races equally, and many of the delusions are more similar than they are different across cultures. How you separate "beliefs" that have no scientific proof from "delusions" that can be defined as pathological is a matter of philosophical debate that will undoubtedly continue over time. It is, however, beyond the scope of this book.

11. What is meant by "positive" and "negative" symptoms?

Positive symptoms are those that produce activity. These are things that are said, acted on, or clearly disturb the individual, such as delusions and hallucinations. **Negative symptoms** (the so-called defect state) are things that are lacking in activity or reduce it—thus "negative." These include a lack of movement, speech, emotional expression, social ability, or initiative to do anything. Positive symptoms tend to fluctuate and respond better to current medications than negative symptoms. Negative symptoms are more stable over time and may be present in the beginning of the illness but are more manifest when the illness becomes chronic and can be the only signs of illness in the stabilized "residual" cases. It is thought that the newer "atypical" medications, such as clozapine, olanzapine, quetiapine, risperidone, and others, may have an effect on reducing negative symptoms. Sometimes depressive symptoms can overlap with negative ones. Since patients with schizophrenia can benefit from antidepressant medication for episodes of depression, these must also be carefully distinguished.

12. Do people with schizophrenia have language problems?

The major symptoms of schizophrenia can all be explained by an underlying disorder in the brain pathways that process language, both that which is perceived and that which is spoken. For example, if the brain hears people speaking to the hearer in an abnormal way so that the connections between the auditory center and brain center meanings in the brain are abnormal, then the hearer will think that something unreal has been said—that is, delusions are then the manifestation. If, on the other hand, an individual is having reflective thoughts about himself or herself but the auditory pathways are misconnected in the brain region that distinguishes what is heard from thoughts, then the thoughts might appear to be actually heard from outside of one's head.

The disorganization of language can more directly be seen as a symptom of these misconnections and can occur in the more severe cases. The negative symptoms of schizophrenia may be either directly caused by language pathway deficits, such as in a lack of complex speech or in a lack of content of speech, or a secondary result of the positive symptoms that are disturbing and preoccupying. Much debate has existed about the relationship of all these symptoms to the primary cause of the illness, but little progress toward a better understanding of the illness has come out of these discussions.

Studies of children who later developed schizophrenia are interesting because some have been shown to have had a delay in the development of language such that the preschizophrenic individual will say his or her first words later than most children and put them into sentences even later. Learning to read is also delayed in these children to a varying degree. This slowing of the acquisition of the building blocks for language suggests abnormalities in the timing and construction of brain pathways for language.

13. Do people with schizophrenia get depression?

Depression is more commonly a characteristic symptom of schizophrenia than most clinicians have realized. In fact, the majority of patients with chronic schizophrenia have had an episode of major depression at some time in the course of their illness. Often the first onset of schizophrenia will be preceded by several months of what patients will describe as a depression.

In addition, as an episode of acute schizophrenia resolves, depression may follow. Sometimes, however, depressive symptoms can be confused with negative symptoms of slowed and less speech, slowed movements, a lack of interest in activities, and general withdrawal (discussed previously). It is when depression can predominate over psychotic symptoms that the diagnosis of schizoaffective disorder or even bipolar disorder might be considered.

14. Are memory problems symptoms of schizophrenia?

Schizophrenia is clearly distinguishable from **Alzheimer's disease**, where recent memory problems are hallmark. A subtle cognitive disturbance, however, is also clearly present in patients with schizophrenia and at an early stage of illness. It is now known from some large research studies that IQ falls somewhat just before the onset of illness and particularly that verbal memory and measures of what is called short-term **"working memory"** are often impaired throughout the illness, although most studies fail to find that these deficits in **cognition** are progressive. They seem to stem from an early brain or adolescent development problem. The nature of the impairment is not known. For example, is it a memory information retrieval problem, as some studies seem to suggest, or an information storage problem? It sometimes is confused with an attention problem. Regardless, people with schizophrenia do not learn new things, particularly of a complex sequential nature, as well as do people without schizophrenia. It is assumed that the cognitive problems stem from structural and thus functional brain disturbances in the frontal and temporal cortices of the brain, particularly on the left side, regions where language is processed. Some medications, such as Cogentin, used to treat the side effects of some of the older neuroleptic medications can have an effect on memory, and this should be taken into account during evaluations of memory problems.

Alzheimer's disease

this is one of a few progressive brain diseases that has been more frequently diagnosed recently in older people who appear disoriented and have difficulty communicating properly with others. It consists of specific characteristic changes in the brain that can be seen only by autopsy after death, but MRI scans can also be revealing.

Working memory

this is a more contemporary term for short-term memory.

Cognition

the quality of the mind that allows animals to think, reason, and manipulate their environment to survive. Cognition can be measured by psychological tests. Of course, the tests are much simpler for nonhuman animals and are most complicated for humans. The well-known IQ is one measure of human cognition.

Characteristics

15. Do people with schizophrenia have a low IQ?

Most individuals with schizophrenia have normal intelligence; however, there is a drop in each individual's IQ at the beginning of illness. Some studies show that individuals with high IQs have a better overall outcome of a schizophrenic episode than people with lower IQs and thus are somewhat protected. In contrast, however, some mental retardation syndromes do co-occur with schizophrenia and, when present, may give clues to the origin of the disorder in those individuals. Usually the latter cases have very poor premorbid histories, the individuals having been educated in special classes in childhood and administered many treatments before adolescence.

16. Are muscular problems associated with schizophrenia?

It used to be thought that any motor problems present in people with schizophrenia, such as the well-known severe example of tardive **dyskinesia**, were a consequence of medications. It is now recognized, and was many decades ago, that some motor disturbance and strange movements known as dyskinesias are present in patients as they are becoming ill and before they took any medications. In fact, some studies show that motor development is somewhat delayed during early childhood in people who later develop schizophrenia (age at first walking), and even at birth some abnormal clumsy movements were detected by one investigator (Elaine Walker, Atlanta) in some now-famous home movies.

Dyskinesia
difficulty in performing movements voluntarily.

17. Do people with schizophrenia have a reduced life span or die from their illness?

It is doubtful that schizophrenia directly reduces the life span. There are even debates as to whether incidences of certain cancers are more rare among people with schizophrenia than in the general population. If you study large populations, however, the age at death might be lower in people with schizophrenia because of proneness to accidents and increased suicide rates, as well as chronic institutionalization in the past that may have led to a lack of rigorous health care and proper nutrition. Still today people with schizophrenia tend not to obtain the adequate healthcare and preventive dietary and health-related measures that can work toward increasing one's life span.

18. Are there medical conditions that look like schizophrenia?

Countless other illnesses are sometimes accompanied by hallucinations and delusions, from metabolic disturbances influencing the brain to viral illnesses, brain tumors, and specific chromosomal abnormalities. The specific aspect of the auditory hallucinations, however, might be different. For example, more than one voice talking about the subject or one voice commenting on the subject's actions is more specific to schizophrenia. The course of illness is more characteristic as well and can be an indication. All the other mentioned causes have other physical symptoms accompanying the psychosis that is uncharacteristic of schizophrenia. When someone presents to a physician with what appears to be a first episode of schizophrenia, good medical practice indicates that these other conditions should be excluded, particularly if there is any indication that they might be present or the characteristics that are seen on the first episode are in any way atypical.

Fertility

having the normal biology that gives one the ability to bear children.

Fecundity

bearing children.

19. Do people with schizophrenia have fewer offspring?

Fertility and **fecundity** are two different entities. People with schizophrenia, if withdrawn and behaviorally different, may not want mates and may not appear attractive to others. Their difficulties in forming close relations generalize to sexual problems as well. This is truer of males than of females, and thus, some studies show that the number of offspring of males with schizophrenia is less than females. Thus, why is an illness that leads to reduced offspring not decreasing? Although in some diseases that continue despite reduced or nonexistent fertility, a genetic advantage is associated with the disadvantageous illness (such as in the case of **sickle-cell anemia** and protection from malaria), no such relationship has been described for schizophrenia. Thus, why schizophrenia still exists today and is not declining in incidence is still unclear and a curious question for researchers to explore.

Sickle-cell anemia

an inherited disease in which the red blood cells, normally disc-shaped, become crescent shaped.

20. Are there some societies in which no individuals develop schizophrenia?

This is a hotly debated issue. E. Fuller Torrey (1980), in his book *Schizophrenia and Civilization*, described pockets of schizophrenia throughout the world and some isolated areas where it is nonexistent. He particularly described the highlands of Papua New Guinea as one region without evidence of schizophrenia. Currently, however, psychiatrists now practicing in Papua New Guinea say that Torrey certainly missed some cases, and documents of such cases do exist in the literature. It would be interesting to study these societies closer. For example, the San tribe of South Africa is said to be the oldest African group in existence; it has isolated itself from society, maintaining its prehistoric hunter–gather culture despite the surrounding civilization. Although there is some indication that schizophrenia does exist among these people, because of tribal laws, it has been difficult for Western-trained professionals to enter their communities to examine whether mental illness exists within the context of their culture. Despite these rare mentioned examples, the World Health Organization has conducted studies over the years to show that schizophrenia is a disease of humanity and is universal. This fact alone may give clues to its genetic origin. A new gene mutation would

Homo sapiens

the scientific desig-
nation for modern
human beings.

Gene

a functional unit of
heredity that is in a
fixed place in the
structure of a chro-
mosome.

be very unlikely to cause schizophrenia, as modern **Homo sapiens** were derived from one bottleneck formed in Africa approximately 150,000 years ago. For a genetic disorder to be universal, it must be as old as modern humans themselves. Since the capacity for complex language is distinctly human and schizophrenia can be seen as a disorder of the biologic pathways for language, a **gene** or genes that define the capacity for language may somehow be related to schizophrenia (Crow, 1997; DeLisi, 2001).

Part Two

Treatment: When, Where, by Whom, and with What?

"In the midst of this godless kneeling, I suddenly remembered that I
had forgotten to take my lithium. . . . I reached into my purse for
my medication, opened the bottle and immediately dropped all of
the pills onto the cathedral floor. The floor was filthy, there were
people all around, and I was too embarrassed to bend over and pick
up the pills."

Kay Redfield Jamison on a trip to Canterbury Cathedral
from her autobiographical revelations about her bouts
with psychiatric illness.

21. What type of professional can treat the first symptoms of schizophrenia?

Many types of doctors and therapists are currently treating the first symptoms of schizophrenia, and because of the types of health services in the United States and other similar countries, the general practitioner, family physician, pediatrician, or emergency room doctor will likely be the first to identify the symptoms. Since the early warning signs can sometimes be indistinguishable from adolescent mood changes, general practitioners and pediatricians will often suggest that the patients will "grow out of it" and that parental controls are necessary.

Many cases have been made public of severely disturbed adolescents whose families and healthcare professionals, initially aware of their behavior, did not understand that an impending psychosis could be approaching. The Columbine High School murders in Colorado were certainly an example. The parents and teachers seemed largely unaware that delusional and bizarre changes were taking place in the boys who had paired together out of common extreme thoughts and interests. They were saying things and acting in a manner that those around them should have been able to detect as serious pathology that was brewing. Instead, they had been in a juvenile detention program and actually had social workers who did not notice their downward spiraling. Several such school incidences have since been reported in the news. The lack of proper identification of those first symptoms before they become a devastating crisis and harmful to other people or themselves is common. Another famous occurrence, the "Long Island Railroad Massacre," was caused by a young adult who for several months became increasingly paranoid and delusional, but his symptoms remained unrecognized by all around him until he boarded a commuter train one evening from Penn Station, New York, with a rifle and shot several passengers randomly.

Although general nonpsychiatric doctors may end up treating people with early schizophrenia, the best treatment will certainly be from trained psychiatrists who are versed in the early signs and latest medications, their doses, efficacy, and side effects and when and how long to medicate. In addition, specifically trained psychiatrists are knowledgeable about providing the needed follow-up and long-term care. This is of course the ideal situation, recognizing that many people with schizophrenia in the United States may quickly use up their health insurance benefits or not be covered at all. The medications are expensive, as is the continued care, and people with schizophrenia tend not to obtain high-paying employment or maintain regular jobs with benefits. In fact, during the prodromal stage, which often lasts a couple of years, it is not uncommon for an individual to lose a job or drop out of college and thus forfeit insurance benefits.

22. Does a psychiatrist always need to be seen and how frequently?

Although general practitioners, psychologists, and social workers who all practice psychotherapy may deal with patients with schizophrenia in their practice, psychiatrists (as stated previously here) know how to use the latest treatment. **Pharmacotherapy** is the primary treatment modality and is only prescribed through a psychiatrist. Although other therapies given by social workers, psychologists, or nurse practitioners can help, such as supportive psychotherapy, **cognitive behavioral therapy** (CBT) family therapy, and orthomolecular therapy (vitamin and mineral treatments), *only* pharmacotherapy will relieve the symptoms. The others are only supplements to medication. Even so, pharmacotherapy does not have all the answers; for example, some patients do not respond well to medications and may even have uncomfortable side effects. Medications do not yet "cure" the actual biological basis for the illness but are likely to be effective for

Pharmacotherapy

treatment of disease through the use of drugs.

Cognitive behavioral therapy (CBT)

this is a brief form of psychotherapy based on the principle that the way one thinks about something causes actions. Thus, it is focused on changing thinking patterns that lead to disruptive behavior.

suppressing the symptoms, much like aspirin suppresses the fever and headache from influenza.

After a patient is stabilized on medication, the psychotherapist, social workers, and occupational therapists need to take a role in providing the social treatments that are needed to improve the quality of life of people with schizophrenia. Rarely will a psychiatrist, who has many patients on his or her rolls, have or take the time to follow up on a patient's practical needs or to make sure that the patient complies with the proper medication regime and other services. The role of other professionals is essential for the support necessary to achieve a favorable outcome for the illness of each patient.

23. Why do some psychiatrists not treat people with schizophrenia?

The average clinical psychiatrist rarely treats people with schizophrenia, at least in the United States, for several reasons. The first is that doctors fear liability from lawsuits if the patient does something harmful to himself or herself or others. These clinicians fear the violence and aggression toward themselves when they frequently practice in isolated private office settings. The second is that people with schizophrenia have limited resources and are almost always unemployed on a regular basis. The nature of their illness means that they will have difficulty working and have no insurance coverage. Even when patients come from families with considerable financial security, they can quickly drain parental savings. Psychiatrists in private practice can rarely see patients with schizophrenia and maintain a livelihood. Thus, these patients are generally seen in clinics by physicians/psychiatrists who have large caseloads and are then followed up by caseworkers and psychiatric social workers. Unfortunately, many people with schizophrenia never make it into a stable treatment setting and are lost to follow-up either after hospitalizations for acute episodes or because they leave the security of a parental home with support and wander away aimlessly, sometimes living on the street as a result of the symptoms.

24. What if I do not have insurance or if my policy does not cover psychiatric care?

Although a lack of insurance is clearly a serious problem with health care today in America and some other countries, the current system is not hopeless. Some public hospital emergency rooms will provide acute care and then make referrals to the appropriate clinic. The social worker assigned to the emergency room often knows what is available in your area. In addition, there are sliding pay scales and many kind-hearted psychiatrists who will not allow the patient to pay more than he or she can afford, although admittedly these people are far too few. Many psychiatrists are now lobbying the U.S. federal government for "parity in health care" for mental illness. Congress must recognize that schizophrenia and other psychiatric disorders are medical illnesses that warrant coverage that is equal to diabetes, hypertension, and other chronic illnesses. Currently, this is not the case, and it has been difficult to get Congress to bring such a bill onto the floor of the House and Senate. Another way to find appropriate healthcare services is to find the nearest local National Alliance for the Mentally Ill (NAMI) chapter. NAMI will have knowledge of the best places to go for immediate treatment and will be able to give advice based on experience often with their own family members. They serve not only as a resource in difficult times but as important continued support for people dealing with mental illness in their families.

25. Do I have to be treated in a hospital if I have schizophrenia and, if so, for how long?

Often, unfortunately, the first time that someone's symptoms of schizophrenia are noticed is when he or she is psychotic (no awareness of reality to the point that they could be harmful to themselves or others). In this case, patients rarely volunteer to go to a hospital and are either forcefully brought there by family or friends, or picked up by the police. In many countries, particularly in impoverished nations, the progress in modernizing hospitals is far behind the Western world, and the reputation of psychiatric hospitals is such that after someone is placed there, he or she is thought to disappear and not come back. There is thus a terrible fear of psychiatric "institutions." Often the hospitals are so ill equipped and ill staffed that they become more of a way to isolate people from society rather than a facility for humanely treating patients with the latest medications. For example, such was the case when I went to visit the National Psychiatric Hospital in El Salvador. It surprised me that even the library where psychiatrists should be able to get the latest advice was void of major journals. Only outdated copies of *The American Journal of Psychiatry* from 10 years ago were on the shelves. In other countries, such as within central Africa, relatives keep afflicted individuals locked in chains to walls or doorknobs of homes in order to keep them from harming themselves or other people. Much publicity occurred many years ago about the conditions of psychiatric hospitals in America, and these were material for Hollywood movies such as *The Snake Pit* that I viewed as a child or *One Flew over the Cuckoo's Nest* from the 1960s. Truthfully, many years ago lobotomies were practiced as the latter movie depicts, and patients lived in squalor as in *The Snake Pit*. Times, however, have clearly changed. Most general hospitals in the United States and other industrialized nations have psychiatry wards, and patients with schizophrenia are kept only as long as required to be stabilized on medication and get into proper longer term outpatient treatment (usually 10 to 30 days).

26. What treatments were used before pharmaceutical companies introduced neuroleptic medication?

The history of treatment for schizophrenia is interesting and is available in several very readable books, although many espouse the authors' prejudices against psychiatry more than relay the facts (Fink, 1999; Whitaker, 2002). A recent best-selling novel in the United Kindom, *Human Traces* (by Sebastian Faulks) gives an interesting historical account of the treatment of people with mental illness over a century ago; but unfortunately this book strays somewhat from the truth when it endows its psychiatrists with the creative hypotheses about the uniquely human nature of schizophrenia that were formulated a century later (Crow, 1997).

People with the symptoms of schizophrenia have always stood out in society as not belonging because of the extreme oddness in the way they look or act. Thus, they have often been dubbed with the terms of "crazy," "loco," "mad," etc. During the late 1800s to the early 20th century and even before, there was a big movement in America and Europe to create large psychiatric institutions to house these individuals and place them far from urban areas. This focus on the question of management of the mentally ill led some to believe that schizophrenia was actually increasing in epidemic proportions throughout Western civilization (Torrey and Miller, 2000), although most researchers believe that this illusion has no scientific basis but rather is due to changes in diagnostic systems and definitions of **insanity**.

Much of the treatment during these times was primarily isolation from society. Various therapies were given, however, including restraints, such as chaining, packing in ice, bloodletting, and even tooth removal. Most hospital wards had not only baths for placing people in cold-packs through a great part of the 20th

Insanity

mental malfunctioning or unsoundness of mind to produce lack of judgment and to the degree that the individual cannot determine right from wrong.

century, but also isolation rooms on every ward so that agitated patients could be taken away from the rest of the patients and staff. Often patients were in these rooms for longer than necessary because of the staff's fear. On some rare occasions, patients who may have been misdiagnosed and were withdrawing from addictive drugs or had cardiac problems unfortunately died while in this kind of therapy. Insulin shock therapy was a popular treatment. One drug, a forerunner of the neuroleptics, was reserpine and was used frequently until phenothiazines became widespread.

In addition, by the mid 20th century, psychoanalysis for schizophrenia became popular and was practiced well into the 1970s in some famous institutions for the well to do—that is, the Menninger Clinic in Kansas and Chestnut Lodge in Maryland. Chestnut Lodge, a beautifully situated campus with lavish rooms and dining facilities and a lovely swimming pool for patient exercise, exposed people to the therapies developed by the well-known analyst Frieda-Fromm Reichman and became popularized by the novel *I Never Promised You a Rose Garden*. Patients were said to need psychoanalytic regression back to infancy and then mothering again through the stages of development slowly for symptomatic improvement and regaining a proper sense of reality. In the 1980s Chestnut Lodge was threatened with losing its accreditation unless neuroleptics were reinstated in the treatment regime for all patients with schizophrenia, and thus, the institution gradually lost the attraction it once had for wealthy families of affected individuals. It fell into disrepute and eventually closed.

27. What about lobotomies?

In the early part of the 20th century, Egas Moniz in Portugal developed a new technique (for which he received the Nobel Prize in Medicine) called "leukotomy." This surgical procedure involved drilling holes in the skull above the temporal lobes and then with the use of a needle-like instrument disrupting connections in brain tissue from several regions of the frontal lobes. This procedure was reported to alleviate the anxiety, agitation, and uncontrollable psychological stress of severely ill institutionalized mental patients. Shortly afterward, Freedman adopted this technique in the United States and performed a few thousand leukotomies (renamed "**lobotomy**") in many patients during the peak of its popularity in the mid 1900s (El-Hai, 2005).

From the late 1930s through the 1950s, lobotomies were widely accepted as good practice in psychiatry throughout the mental hospitals in the United States. Although some individuals were dramatically helped by this procedure, there was also much abuse of its use, extending the indications for lobotomies to patients who the nursing staff simply found "difficult" and behavioral problems in the social setting of institutional life. Even the very wealthy and well-connected families (as in the famous case of the Kennedys' daughter) had lobotomies performed unscrupulously on affected family members.

28. What are the choices for medication?

Since the 1960s, **antipsychotic** medication has been the mainstay treatment for schizophrenia, and the outcome is better if individuals with schizophrenia receive this treatment early in the course of the illness. In fact, it has been said that the new medications "emptied" the psychiatric hospitals of the long-term patients in the 1960's and brought people with schizophrenia into the mainstream of society. Severe variable side effects of these medications still existed, however, and doses went higher and higher to achieve clinical effect. Many patients still did not respond even to very high doses. In the 1970s, clozapine was introduced in Europe and was a drug that had remarkable effects in patients who did not respond to the usual medications. However, when cases were reported of life-threatening

Lobotomy
the surgical division of one or more brain tracts. It is usually referred to as cutting nerves that run from the frontal lobe to the thalamus in the brain. It has been done in various ways, most often by inserting a needle above the nose in between the eyes. This serves to disconnect nerves connecting the frontal lobe of the brain to other structures.

Antipsychotic
any medication that specifically suppresses the positive symptoms of hallucinations and delusions. This medication can also be useful in other conditions as a strong tranquilizer.

leucopenia caused by clozapine and in rare instances when some patients died, its use was limited and not placed on the market in the United States. By the late 1980s, however, there was renewed interest in clozapine in the United States, and reports were making the newspapers of miraculous recoveries of individuals who were completely psychotic and thought disordered before clozapine, and then becoming normal, well groomed, released from the hospital, and applying for employment on the drug. New trials were begun in the United States, and the FDA approved the use of clozapine for treatment of patients with tardive dyskinesia, as it appeared not to lead to this serious side effect. It was also approved for patients who were nonresponsive to other medications. The disadvantage was that these individuals taking clozapine had to be followed closely with blood testing on a frequent basis to assure that they did not develop blood dyscrasias, such as the leucopenia seen in the past. It was later noted that clozapine seemed to have a unique effect on preventing suicidal tendencies. Thus, its value today as a primary treatment for schizophrenia should not be overlooked. No cases of serious leukopenia or deaths have been reported since its reinstitution.

In the meantime, many pharmaceutical companies have been developing new drugs for schizophrenia that have similar neurochemical mechanisms to clozapine but are less toxic to the blood system. Several of these have now reached the market and have been used for the last decade. They have been dubbed the second-generation neuroleptics, or "atypicals," and include the Janssen Pharmaceuticals drug Risperdal (risperidone), the Lilly drug Zyprexa (olanzapine), Astra-Zeneca drug Seroquel (quetiapine), Bristol-Myers Squibb Abilify (aripiprazole), and the Pfizer drug Geodon (ziprasidone). Doses and potency vary among these drugs, but in general they have the same efficacy, much lower incidence of side effects, and thus good tolerability compared with the earlier generation of drugs such as Haldol, Thorazine, Mellaril, Navane, and others.

29. What are the medication side effects?

The two side effects of the atypicals that have received a lot of publicity are substantial weight gain, more so with Zyprexa than with the other drugs, and diabetic-like problems with glucose metabolism. Although each drug company will report studies indicating that their drug has less side effects than those of their competitors and in many areas more efficacy, it is hard to tease out the bias in this reporting. Thus, the NIMH invested funds in a large multicenter comparison trial called CATIE using several of these drugs and one of the older drugs as well to compare their efficacy and side effects. Suprisingly, little differences between the drugs have emerged in the initial stages of data analyses, but more results will be reported soon.

The older drugs, such as Haldol, Thorazine, and others, have not been used much in the United States over the past few years because the efficacy of the atypicals has been clearly proven. However, some other countries still predominantly use them, and thus, motor side effects can still be seen. Mainly the old medications produced Parkinsonian-like side effects (tremors and stiffness), and in some cases, tardive dyskinesia was a particularly severe side effect of pronounced uncontrollable motor movements of the limbs and tongue. With the discontinuation of medication, sometimes it was reversible, but often not. Also, trials of discontinuation and then reinstitution of the medications often made tardive dyskinesia even worse. This debilitating condition was widely feared, not only because of the disability it caused but also because of the peculiar look it gave its victims, forcing them to stand out in public and be stigmatized. Other side effects included sedation, dizziness, hypotension, a lack of sexual drive, and hepatic damage. None of these side effects appears to be a concern for the newer second-generation antipsychotics.

30. What are the treatments for side effects?

Some medications such as Cogentin and Artane (anticholinergic and antihistaminic) are used solely for the tremors and stiffness, but despite these, most patients on those older drugs had visible effects. There are now new treatments currently being developed for the weight gain and the metabolic effects of the new atypical drugs.

31. Are there alternative treatments to medication?

I do not believe that there are alternatives to medications, and the advertisements for so-called alternatives are misleading. There are only supplementary treatments, some of which have no effect, such as vitamins and dietary supplements, and others that may have some modest effect, such as CBT.

32. What is cognitive behavioral therapy?

CBT has become a popular treatment for many emotional and behavioral traits. For schizophrenia, it has recently become a popular adjunct to medication at a time when the patient is stabilized but has a baseline of functional disturbances that are not alleviated by medication. In addition, one study in Manchester, England, claims effects on delaying the onset of schizophrenia by treatment with CBT alone during the **prodrome**. This finding, however, remains to be replicated. Several carefully performed research studies have documented its efficacy, and this treatment is particularly frequently used in the United Kingdom, although also by some psychologists in the United States as well.

CBT has two components: behavioral and cognitive. Behavior therapy is supposed to weaken the connec-

Prodrome

an early or premonitory symptom of a disease. If true specific prodromal symptoms are known, one can detect the illness early. These symptoms signify that the disease will be almost certain.

tions between troublesome situations and an individual's reactions to them. The reactions are such emotions as fear, depression, or rage and other self-defeating or self-damaging behavior. The cognitive aspect of the therapy focuses on changing thought patterns in order to change the emotional state and thus behavior. CBT has been used successfully in conditions such as depression, panic or anxiety disorders, and phobias. The basis for CBT in schizophrenia is that the disorder consists of a circumscribed set of irrational beliefs, and thus easily learned techniques can alleviate the impact of those beliefs on one's daily life. The CBT therapists work to make patients aware that their thinking patterns are distorted and then train them to change these patterns by a process called "cognitive restructuring." This is different from psychodynamic psychotherapy, which instead tries to make patients understand why they behave the way they do and assumes that with understanding comes change. CBT does not involve understanding why one behaves a certain way but uses behavior modification techniques to produce change in behavior. Some of these techniques include behavioral homework assignments that encourage patients to try new responses to difficult situations. Another is called "cognitive rehearsal," where a patient imagines a difficult situation and the therapist guides him or her through dealing with it. Patients may also keep a journal of their thoughts, feelings, and actions, although this may be difficult for patients with schizophrenia. The therapist also will use conditioning (positive reinforcement) and systematic desensitization from fears. Treatment is relatively short in comparison to some other forms of psychotherapy, usually lasting no longer than 16 weeks. Although many insurance plans provide reimbursement for cognitive-behavioral therapy services, they may not yet reimburse for this treatment in schizophrenia. Several organizations specialize in CBT in the United States (Albert Ellis Institute [formerly the Institute for Rational-Emotive Therapy]; 45 East 65th Street, New York, NY 10021, 1-800-323-4738, http://www.rebt.org; Beck Institute, GSB Building, City Line and Belmont Avenues, Suite 700, Bala Cynwyd, PA 19004-1610, 1-610-664-3020, http://www.beckinstitute.org; and the National Association of Cognitive-Behavioral Therapists, P.O. Box 2195, Weirton, WV 26062, 1-800-853-1135, http://www.nacbt.org). In the United Kingdom, Dr. Douglas Turkington at the University of Newcastle upon Tyne and Dr. Til Wykes at the Institute of Psychiatry in London, as well as others, have written books on this topic (e.g. Turkington & Turkington, 1995; Reeder and Wykes, 2005).

33. Can a specific diet help?

Unfortunately, throughout the years, there have been proponents of the idea that something in the diet (e.g., too much sugar, aspartame, and pesticides sprayed on field-grown food, as well as not enough **fish oils**) could cause schizophrenia. Popular organizations stressed that dietary changes would rid the body of toxins, and they encouraged patients with schizophrenia, unfortunately, to discontinue neuroleptic medications. Families would often turn to these organizations, particularly when their relative was in a particularly severe state and control by medication was difficult. These organizations have been dangerous because they propose plans that have not been substantiated by rigorous research studies or treatment trials. You can today find many websites that encourage these alternative treatments.

34. What about vitamins and fish oil?

Celebrities, who serve as role models, unfortunately are also prone to trying these unconventional treatments and publicize them (e.g., Margot Kidder, the movie star who acted in the Superman series). Margot had a severe highly publicized psychotic episode several years ago that led her to become homeless for a while. She claims that medications were not the

Fish oil

3-Omega fatty acids. These are substances important for the building of the lining of nerves. For good functioning of the nervous system, it is important that these fatty acids are in abundance. This is a commercial product that can be bought in health food stores at various levels of purity and has been advertised as a "cure-all" for many conditions; most claims have not been substantiated scientifically.

answer for her. Recently, she appeared on a well-known television talk show recounting how vitamin and mineral therapies have made her symptom free and that Dr. Hoffer, who introduced her to this, saved her life. Dr. Abram Hoffer is well known for his vitamin cocktails that have never been substantiated with scientific treatment trials. Nevertheless, he maintained a faithful following for many years in Saskatchewan, Canada. Large does of vitamin B3 (niacin) are the mainstay of his treatment. This is based on the knowledge that niacin is converted to nicotinamide adenine dinucleotide, an important coenzyme for facilitating various metabolic processes in the body. Niacin also has antihistaminic (antiallergen) properties. Thus, Hoffer's assumption is that "brain allergies" are responsible to some degree for schizophrenic behavior. Part of his regime is a reduced sugar and junk-food diet, which he says requires more niacin to metabolize. He also claims that schizophrenic patients make a substance in their brain that serves as an endogenous hallucinogen and that niacin serves to reduce this toxin in the body. To summarize, no scientific studies can substantiate any of Dr. Hoffer's claims, and in general, for people with schizophrenia, he does more harm than good in espousing and writing books about the merits of this treatment regime.

Another recognized pioneer in this field was David Horobin, who recently died. His area of research had been the clinical use of gamma-linolenic acid (GLA), an omega-3 derivative of an essential oil. It is present in the evening primrose, borage, and black currant seeds. He was one of the first to claim benefits from GLA in treating disease conditions of the nervous system. During his lifetime he founded Scotia Pharmaceuticals and later Laxdale, Ltd. in Scotland and the journals *Medical Hypotheses* and *Prostaglandins, Leukotrienes,* and *Essential Fatty Acids.* He was an energetic promoter of evening primrose oil in the treatment of schizophrenia and represented his company in campaigning vigorously for senior renowned scientists to conduct trials of its use. To date, some small studies suggest that it might be weakly beneficial as an adjunct to conventional medication in persons who do not completely respond to their normal treatment regime. Many studies fail to find such an effect. His own controversial trials were under way at the time that he developed a malignant lymphoma from which he died in 2003. He was an extremely engaging and convincing personality, who has had little following to explore his hypotheses further since his untimely death.

35. Can psychotherapy help?

Psychotherapy

the treatment of mental or emotional problems by psychological means.

Many types of **psychotherapy** are available. The major reason for someone to consider psychotherapy is that he or she fails to be able to help himself or herself to make progress functioning satisfactorily with family and friends and in an occupation and would like to improve the quality of life. People with schizophrenia benefit most from help with practical issues. Group therapy can be not only a helpful mechanism to improve one's condition but a social measure as well. The most useful type of therapy to these patients supplements long-term neuroleptic medication and guides the patient in strengthening the complexity of his or her daily activities. Learning how to reach attainable goals through positive reinforcement and encouragement is far more useful than insight-oriented psychodynamic therapy, which is more important for nonpsychotic individuals. Often this therapeutic setting can be provided best by psychiatric social workers.

36. Can family therapy help?

Family therapy

any of several therapeutic approaches in which a family is treated as a whole.

Family therapy grew out of the many psychodynamic treatments that reached their peak in the 1970s. Two main principles were involved: the first is that there were communication disturbances within the family that led to confusion in the affected individual and which resulted in the symptoms of schizophrenia, and the second is that the patient is not the individual brought for treatment but rather the family unit as a whole. In general, the family therapy movement has caused a lot of damage to the well-being of families and to the relationship between the caregivers and consumers. Parents were told (or at least it was implied) that they were somehow at fault, and they did not want to be blamed. They needed help to deal with all the management issues that occur when a family member has a serious mental illness. This thus strained the relationship between families and the medical community, and it has taken many years to regain the trust that is needed for families to support the pharmacotherapy that is essential to treat those individuals with schizophrenia.

37. How long does medication have to be taken?

Taking medication for schizophrenia is similar to taking medication for high blood pressure. Although someone who has only one episode of a psychosis should have a closely monitored trial without medications after they are free of symptoms for one year, in 90 percent of these cases, the illness does reoccur within the first five years. Thus, treatment is generally long term and is considered necessary for the first decade after symptoms have appeared. If some symptoms, even residual negative ones, are still apparent, medication should be taken indefinitely. With recovery, the medication can be slowly tapered after several years and stopped. Not enough research is yet available to determine how long people need to take preventive medication and who will not benefit from a lifetime of medications.

38. Is electroconvulsive therapy used for schizophrenia?

Electroconvulsive therapy

a type of treatment usually for depression that gives a series of electrical shocks to regions of the brain given in sessions that are separated by several days. The way it exerts its effects is unknown. However, it is not dangerous or painful and is accompanied by an anesthetic when administered. The only known side effect is memory loss subsequent to the treatment.

Electroconvulsive therapy (ECT) has received bad press over the years for both its treatment in schizophrenia and also depression. Some hospitals do not allow it, and doctors' privileges to use it are separate from their regular medical licenses and hospital privileges. Certainly, if this is a recommended treatment, the qualifications for the person performing the ECT should be researched. This is a procedure that with anticonvulsant medication given at the same time is actually quite safe. Controversy exists, however, as to its efficacy for schizophrenia. Most studies do not show clear long-term results and certainly do not prevent the patient from having a recurrence even if the acute episode subsides. Maintenance antipsychotic medication will then need to be given. However, one of the reasons to give ECT rather than antipsychotic medication as the first treatment of choice is to avoid the side effects of medication. This is less of an issue now with the advent of the newer medications that have relatively minimal side effects. One side effect of ECT is memory loss, and whether this loss is permanent is unclear. ECT is more commonly given as the last resort in patients with schizophrenia when they have particularly comorbid depressive, manic, or violent symptoms that do not respond to usual medications. Max Fink (1999), a well-known authority on ECT, has written a helpful book about its uses. In it he describes the beneficial effect of ECT for what he calls "the thought disorders"—the delusional and hallucinatory and language disorganization symptoms that occur predominantly in schizophrenia, but also in other illnesses as well. The number of ECT treatments (as many as 15 to 25), however, that is needed to alleviate these symptoms is larger than that for depression, and it may take longer for the ECT to reach its effect. In addition, if a course of ECT is not repeated, then relapse often occurs. A minimum of six months of treatment is recommended (Fink, 1999). The failure of ECT for schizophrenia that psychiatrists and families conclude could rather be due to a lack of continuation of the treatment than a lack of its usefulness. A combination of ECT and antipsychotic medication may be more efficacious than either alone. Dr. Fink describes the mechanism as one in which the ECT can increase the ability for the medication to enter the neuronal cell membranes and thus exert its physiologic effect. The patient then might also require a smaller dose of the medication and be less likely to experience its side effects. Nevertheless, few psychiatrists use ECT today for schizophrenia, and they are generally not trained to do so in their medical school residencies.

39. What are the pros and cons of participating in research studies?

Many of the major academic institutions have psychiatrists who conduct research on schizophrenia. Currently, relatively little is known about this disease compared with most other medical disorders; thus, research of multiple kinds needs to continue, with adequate funding from public sources. Although many theories about schizophrenia exist, the fact still is that there is no biological test for it, there are no symptoms that are specific to schizophrenia, and there is no preventive measure one can take to avoid getting this illness. We only know that it has an inherited component of some sort and that it appears usually in early adulthood or late adolescence, that it has some sex differences, and that medications can suppress the symptoms, such as having delusionary perceptions and auditory hallucinations, as long as these medications are taken continuously as prescribed. Research is desperately needed to find drugs that target the cause of illness and to find treatments that prevent the chronic course before it begins. Participating in research studies generally does not help the individual directly but can, in the future, benefit others who develop the illness. Often, however, being in a research study means, generally, that better care is available to oneself and one's family because the researchers are generally well recognized as experts in their field and will know where and how to obtain the best treatment, although this is not always the case. Access to care is then facilitated, and earlier detection may result for other family members that can lead then to a better outcome. The NIMH often lists various research studies on their website. Researchers advertise through clinics, hospitals, and support groups such as NAMI so that if you would like to be a part of some of these studies that are generally not risky this should be possible.

Part Three

The Consideration of Nongenetic Risk Factors

"*The mystique of science proclaims that numbers are the ultimate test of objectivity. Surely we can weigh a brain or score an intelligence test without recording our social preferences. If ranks are displayed in hard numbers obtained by rigorous and standardized procedures, then they must reflect reality, even if they confirm what we want to believe from the start. . . . If quantitative data are as subject to cultural constraint as any other aspect of science, then they have no special claim upon final truth.*"

Steven Jay Gould, *The Mismeasure of Man*, 1981

40. Do birth complications cause schizophrenia?

Numerous studies on the association of obstetric complications (both **prenatal** and perinatal) with schizophrenia have been reported over the years. No single specific complication has been implicated, however. These are a summation of various things, such as bleeding during pregnancy, influenza during the second trimester, premature birth, and excessively long labor. Some investigators have hypothesized that many birth complications lead to transient hypoxia to the developing brain, and when occurring at a particular stage in development, the later fully developed brain will be more vulnerable to schizophrenia. Particularly, it is thought that the cells of the **hippocampus** are most vulnerable to perinatal complications, such that its growth may be suppressed during a crucial time period. These are just theories without proof, and in fact, however, some good studies exist that now show no association of later schizophrenia with having been born with birth complications. At least one study of siblings with and without schizophrenia shows that they have no difference in frequency of having had birth complications. Thus, how can one draw conclusions about these data? First, the studies examining birth complications use various methods for selecting control individuals for comparison and for obtaining a history of birth complications. Controls need to be matched for social class and sex. When this is done by comparison to well siblings for an example, then the association with birth complications is less clear. Similarly, taking an obstetric history from mothers is fraught with subjectiveness, as it has been shown that mothers tend to remember more birth complications occurring in their chronically ill offspring than those who are well. Thus, the stronger studies are those that are prospective analyses of large birth cohorts where data have been archived systematically from birth. Several of these in the United Kingdom and United States have been published with equivocal results over-

Prenatal

the period between conception and birth.

Hippocampus

this relatively small brain structure lies deep within the temporal lobe and is thought to be crucial for memory. It has been given this name because of its unusual shape.

all. Given that the vast majority of adults who have a history of prenatal complications *do not* develop schizophrenia, it is suspected that these are not significant risk factors for schizophrenia. Mothers who suffer such complications should not have to worry that in the future their offspring will be any more likely to develop schizophrenia than their peers. Pediatricians should not be warning of such.

41. Is schizophrenia more common in some cultural or racial groups than others?

The answer to this question is most likely no. Steven J. Gould in his book *Mismeasure of Man* showed that seemingly objective quantitative data can be erroneously shown to be associated with the wrong characteristics due to societal bias, such as in the association of head size and intelligence (see the previous quote). Some studies have associated schizophrenia with lower socioeconomic status, and in some countries, this diagnosis appears more frequently in one racial or cultural group rather than another. The reasons for this are many. First, physicians tend to be more likely to diagnose schizophrenia rather than other forms of psychosis in persons who do not communicate well because their culture or language is different from the physician's or because it is not understood well. For example, in some religious sects in the United States and other countries, services become highly emotional with chanting that can give some people the appearance of being acutely psychotic, as people are "communicating with God." In some cultures, paranoia may be justified given the political history that some individuals have been a part of. The examples can go on. Nevertheless, the World Health Association has conducted multicenter incidence studies to show that schizophrenia is present throughout the world at relatively similar incidence rates across many different cultures. Other reports indicate its presence in Papua New Guinea (despite previous reports to the contrary), the Australian aboriginals, and the isolated ancient San population of South Africa. In fact, schizophrenia is possibly present in every population of the world because its origins are as old as the origins of modern Homo sapiens themselves. One great thinker on schizophrenia (Crow, 1997) describes schizophrenia as "the price Homo sapiens pays for language," meaning that schizophrenia is at the extreme of the uniquely human genetic variation that distinguishes modern human beings from all other primates and gave us the ability to communicate by complex language.

42. Can bad family relationships cause schizophrenia?

An emphatic answer to this question is *no*, and this myth must be dispelled. Several years ago it was popular among psychiatrists and psychologists to presume that the cause of schizophrenia had to do with poor mothering, or the "schizophrenogenic mother," as the term became coined. This was a mother that was supposedly giving mixed messages to her child, causing pathologic ambivalence and confusion. This notion, however, was not based on any carefully controlled research studies, but rather on subjective observations of some senior well-respected psychodynamically oriented psychiatrists of the time. Another set of researchers introduced the term *expressed emotion* to the field and produced data to suggest that the greater the expressed emotion in a family, the more likely a psychosis would develop in an individual. These data, however, were refuted by others who argued that higher expressed emotion in any family with a schizophrenic member may have more to do with the frustration the family feels having to deal with a chronically ill individual who can cause frequent serious crises by virtue of the disorder itself. At best, one can say that a kind, reassuring, protective, and supportive intact family will aid someone afflicted with schizophrenia to have a better outcome to his or her illness than a disruptive and unsupportive family environment.

43. What about immigration from another county?

Some very interesting studies in the United Kingdom and the Netherlands have shown that Afro-Caribbeans and other migrant groups to foreign countries have an increase of schizophrenia in themselves and their offspring after having arrived in a foreign culture. Currently, the cause of this phenomenon is unclear—that is, whether it is genetic or environmental or an artifact of the data collection, but that the difficulties adjusting to life in a foreign country economically and socially can certainly provide fertile ground for the development of all kinds of emotional problems in later life. Despite these reports, the vast majority of immigrants to new lands do not develop schizophrenia. One could comment that countries such as the United States and Australia made up by a majority of different waves of immigrant groups over time have not reported increases in schizophrenia as a result.

44. Is it better to live in a rural area?

Some epidemiologic surveys have found that schizophrenia appears more prevalent in urban than rural areas within the same county. Similarly, the prevalence of schizophrenia may be less, although the incidence the same, in underdeveloped rather than developed industrialized countries. This may be comparable to the urban versus rural distinction. Reasons for this disparity could be many but may have to do with the outcome of acute psychotic episodes. In general, rural and nonindustrialized environments tend to have extended families living together or close by, and thus emotional support for psychotic individuals is greater. These individuals also tend to be tolerated more in these environments and have more space to be alone so that they do not need to interact by force with others. It would be easier to stay out of a hospital or treatment facility existing in such environments. Recovery might be seen as a nonviolent, quiet behavior, and the inner world of someone with schizophrenia would not only be more tolerable but less noticeable. This does not mean, however, that it is better to live in a rural area if you have schizophrenia! Urban environments tend to provide patients with better medical care, more available psychiatrists and related healthcare personnel, and better access to the newest treatments.

45. Is schizophrenia infectious?

Once a curious Russian physician, who reported the results from an epidemiological survey of dwellings in Moscow, claimed that clusters of schizophrenia occurred in specific neighborhoods (Kasanetz, 1979). Torrey (1980) in his book on *Schizophrenia and Civilization* claims that pockets of schizophrenia exist in counties of Ireland, suggesting that schizophrenia could be infectious or spread from one individual to another. Crow and Done (1986), however, in a landmark analysis of a large number of pairs of siblings with schizophrenia showed that despite two siblings living together having schizophrenia, the time of onset of their illness was not correlated, although their age of onset was. If an illness is contagious, one expects that two people living together would get it relatively close in time. If they seem to get the illness at the same age, the onset is predetermined by other factors such as developmental and/or genetic ones. Thus, the infectious theory "holds no water" and has largely been abandoned.

46. Do viruses cause schizophrenia?

An infectious agent may cause an illness, however, without being directly infectious. Dating back to Menninger in the early 1900s, there was a suspicion that viruses could cause schizophrenia. As Karl Menninger noted (1926), the great influenza epidemic of 1918 saw an increase of schizophrenia admissions to hospitals. Through the years since, particularly revived by Torrey and Peterson (1976), the viral hypothesis of schizophrenia has carried weight among some researchers even today. Many viral infections have been implicated besides influenza, such as cytomegalic virus, herpes I and II, Epstein-Barr virus, toxoplasmosis, and some uniquely human retroviruses. The positive findings from these studies, however, have not been consistently replicated, and no active viral particles have ever been definitively isolated from the brains of people with schizophrenia after death. The most prevalent theory about these viruses is that a mother acquires the infection during the second trimester of pregnancy, a crucial time for brain higher cortical center development, and that this makes offspring more vulnerable to develop schizophrenia in later life. This is just a theory that does not yet produce convincing substantiating evidence.

Part Four

The Genetic Risk

"*Mendel had painstakingly backcrossed pollen and egg cells from the common pea plant to reach a better understanding of inheritance. Mendel had recorded . . . his findings in a two-part lecture in 1865 . . . and then was all but ignored for the rest of his life . . ." but rediscovered by Bateson in May 1900. Nearly a century after the debate over Mendelism that set the stage for contemporary genetics, almost every part of our modern understanding of how the world works—the relationship between parent and offspring . . . and the commonalities among all living things—can in a large measure be traced back to that startling spring of 1900, when anything was possible.*"

Robin Marantz Henig (2000), *The Monk in the Garden*

47. What are the lessons from history?

The ideas of "genes," "genetics," and specific patterns
of inheritance grew out of the discoveries of the late
1800s and early 1900s, and thus the field of "genetics"
was born, gradually evolving into what we know of its
science today. With it, however, also grew the notion
of "eugenics" (i.e., that if genetic defects caused unde-
sirable traits, one could eliminate these traits in society). Sterilization became an acceptable procedure for
people who were considered "misfits" in society and
included those with mental retardation and also psychiatric disturbances. Although little is publicized
about these times, the Coldspring Harbor Laborato-
ries (Long Island, New York), today a center of excel-
lence in molecular genetics, was then a "hotbed" in the
United States for the eugenics movement. The Holo-
caust of the mid 20th century looms high on the list of
human atrocities inflicted on our fellow man in recent
times. It was characterized by a program for the extermination of people for the sole reason that their her-
itage included Jewish ancestry. However, less is
publicized about the considerable participation of
German psychiatrists at that time in the extermination
of psychotic patients in psychiatric hospitals. In Ger-
many alone at least five main such hospitals were
equipped with gas chambers and connected incinera-
tors during the years from 1938 to 1940. Preservation
of the building for such procedures can be seen today
in the Hadamar Psychiatric Hospital, a short distance
from Frankfurt, where a museum depicts the scene of
busloads of patients being delivered each day down to
the "showers" by one door and then out the opposite
door as corpses to the autopsy table for the academic
neuropathologist/psychiatrist to have an opportunity
to examine the postmortem brain before incineration.
Eventually, but not before 10,000 patients were exter-
minated in this way at Hadamar, the Bishop of Muen-
ster spoke out about this suspected atrocity, and Hitler
was forced to abandon this effort in the psychiatric
hospitals. Nevertheless, the doctors and nurses continued various methods of euthanasia by injection and

starvation until the end of World War II and the fall of the Nazi party. This is a striking example of the extreme misuse of genetic information. One may simply read this and say that it cannot happen again and that perhaps the lesson from history has been learned. But has it?

We are part of a different scientific age now. The explosion of new technology in the field of genetics has enabled us to have available methods of identifying variations in almost all genes in the human genome. What will be done with this information now that we have it needs continual discussion and legislation. The science fiction movie *Gattaca* produced not long ago is an example of what could go wrong or is wrong. Two classes of human beings were in this movie: those whose genes were "enhanced" in utero (i.e., deleterious variants were replaced with "better" ones) and those individuals who were born of natural unions between men and women. The latter were discriminated against, could not get professional jobs, and were forbidden to marry those who were enhanced. Everyone carried his or her own **DNA** card, which was proof of their identity. Could this happen in reality? Scientifically, no barriers exist. Already in vitro fertilization allows parents to choose the eye and hair color for a baby and unlimited other characteristics of their choice. What we do with new genetic information must be open for serious discussion.

48. Who were the Genain quadruplets?

On April 14, 1930, four identical quadruplets weighing from 3 to 4 pounds 8 ounces were born by natural birth after a short labor and were placed in incubators. Although their childhood achievements varied, they grew up close and with much societal attention until within 6 months of each other in their early adulthood, they all had acute psychotic episodes eventually diagnosed as schizophrenia. Their notoriety as four identical individuals who all had schizophrenia led to their being brought to the NIMH Laboratory of Psychology in the 1950s to be studied by a well-known group of investigators interested in searching for the causes of schizophrenia and particularly in pursuing the gene environment or nature versus nurture controversy. Every test in use at that time, from the Rorschach to conventional **electroencephalograms** (EEGs), was given to the Genains. These investigators, David Rosenthal and Seymour Kety, first director of NIMH, went on from there to design adoption studies to be conducted in Denmark and produced pioneering data that turned the thinking of the time around from environmental to genetic/biological causes. There were also studies of twins at NIMH, such as those studied by David Shakow, who led to many theories about environment and development of people who get schizophrenia. David Rosenthal, however, was the one that particularly developed a relationship with the family of the quadruplets, giving them the name "Genain" meaning "bad blood" and pseudonyms as Nora, Iris, Myrna, and Hester (representing NIMH) so that he could publish his findings but maintain the family's privacy. Again in 1979, after publication of the Kety-Rosenthal adoption studies and international recognition of the implications of these results, the Genains, then age 50, were brought back to NIMH to the laboratory of neuropsychopharmacology, to be examined for abnormalities in all of the biological markers that were claimed to be important for schizophrenia at the time. I was privileged to be a young postdoctoral fellow in charge of managing the procedures and caring for these women during their two-month stay on the inpatient research ward. At that time David Rosenthal accompanied them to NIMH but quickly remained in the background, dealing with his own newly diagnosed Alzheimer's disease. During the period of getting to know these women, their fears, and variety of similar delusions and hallucinations, I also came to know the kind silent face of Dr. Rosenthal, whose personal copy of his book was later taken off his office shelf and presented to me for my

Electroencephalogram (EEG)

a type of test whereby electrodes are placed on several areas of the head and recordings are made of the brain's electrical activity.

service to the Genains in his absence. Whether we learned anything useful from working intensely with the Genains during that period was questionable, but the experience left a deep impression in my memory— no family can have such bad luck as to have four of four children with schizophrenia unless the illness was genetic. My later mentor in psychiatric genetics, Elliot S. Gershon, remarked during that time, when I commented on his lack of investment in our studies of the Genains, that I had gotten myself an "N of one," meaning essentially only one case study, nothing more, because these women all shared the identical DNA sequences, and that nothing fruitful could come out of such a genetic comparison study of any scientific rigor. Of course, he was ahead of the times and was correct, already a pioneer himself in more fruitful genetic research.

49. Is schizophrenia inherited? And if so, how?

The thought that schizophrenia is inherited dates back to early 20th-century descriptions of the condition (*Dementia Praecox* by Emil Kraepelin). He estimated that "defective heredity," as he called it, was prominent and present in over 70 percent of cases (Kraepelin, 1907). From his early writings on, large family studies were conducted throughout Europe, particularly to estimate the amount of illness in close family members of individuals with schizophrenia. In general, they were consistent with the notion that there was an excess risk for schizophrenia to close relatives (siblings, offspring) of approximately 10 percent but that the risks fell dramatically in more distant relatives, such as aunts, uncles, and cousins. The highest risks, however, were shown to be present in **monozygotic twin** pairs based on a series of independent twin studies. The biggest dilemma in psychiatric genetics today, however, is the attempt to explain why, although the risk to monozygotic twins is highest of any recorded risk factor for schizophrenia, it falls considerably short of 100

Monozygotic twins
twins born at the same time who originate from the splitting of the same egg after it has been fertilized. The DNA is identical in both twins; and thus the twins are sometimes referred to as identical.

percent (i.e., only 50 percet on average), which is the percentage you would expect if two individuals share an identical genetic makeup.

Although most people seem to think that this low concordance rate among identical twins is evidence for environmental interactions, modification for gene expression by internally controlled molecular mechanisms has not been excluded. The turning point in schizophrenia research and probably the most important data collection and results of the 20th century in this field came from the carefully planned and executed adoption studies of Seymour Kety and David Rosenthal using Danish case registries to identify parents with schizophrenia and their offspring (Rosenthal and colleagues, 1968) and adopted at birth children who developed schizophrenia, their biological and adoptive relatives (Kety and colleagues, 1968). As a group, regardless of the study design, these investigators showed that an excess of schizophrenia was present in the biological relatives of individuals with schizophrenia, but not the adoptive relatives. These data were fuel for the nature/nurture debates of the time and initiated great changes in the focus of research on schizophrenia from the 1970s to the present. Initially, when these results were reported, the leadership of academic psychiatry departments throughout the United States was predominantly made up of psychoanalysts, and this was true of the most prestigious of training institutes. Soon these individuals, however, were replaced by biologically oriented chairpersons who led a new era of research—and the field of biological psychiatry was born.

50. If my aunt, uncle, or cousin has schizophrenia, what are the chances of my children getting it?

Children would share the same amount of genetic material with a parent's uncle as with their own first cousin (parent's sibling's child), and the risk for schizophrenia in both cases would be very small (Table 1) and almost the same as in the general population.

	A %	B %
Identical twins	48	100
Non-identical twins	17	50
Siblings	9	50
Children	13	50
Parents	6	50
Grandchildren	5	25
Nieces and nephews	4	25
Aunts and uncles	2	25
First cousins	2	12.5
Unrelated individuals	1	1

Table 1. A: Familial risks for schizophrenia in relatives of people with schizophrenia (modified from Gottesman, 1994); B: Risks for a genetic dominant trait

51. If I have a brother with schizophrenia and my partner does too, what are the chances of our children getting schizophrenia?

If the illness is present in both sides of the family, then the chances of a child becoming affected would be greater, although there are no clear statistics to say how much greater. In addition, these are only general risk statistics, and thus what happens in each individual family will vary. We do not know what the real risks are until the actual genes that lead to a predisposition for schizophrenia are identified and their mechanisms for producing disease determined. The risks shown in Table 1 are based only on prevalence rates from the old large family studies that exist. Moreover, one has to consider that since the 1980s there have been newer carefully controlled family studies using the American Psychiatric Association DSM diagnostic categories. In these studies the risk to any close family relative is still in excess but is considerably lower than in previous reports (on average about 7 to 8 percent).

52. If I have an identical twin with schizophrenia, but I am well, what are my children's chances of having schizophrenia?

According to some twin studies, it appears that the risk for schizophrenia to offspring of well versus ill identical twins is the same and would be similar to the risk to children in general (i.e., 13%; Table 1). These studies, however, have been flawed in design and limited in their numbers. People with schizophrenia, particularly men, have fewer offspring than those who do not have schizophrenia; thus, the number of offspring of ill versus well identical twins will not likely be the same. Because of the difficulties in obtaining and studying identical twins where one has schizophrenia, the numbers for comparisons in these studies are small. This issue is thus still controversial but is an important one. If these rates were equal, then one assumes that something in the genetic sequence (identical DNA sequence) must be what is crucial for schizophrenia susceptibility. If these rates really are unequal, *although* still in excess in the offspring of the well co-twin, then some modification of the defective gene's expression, either endogenously or by the environment, is likely to be taking place as well. We hope that molecular genetic studies of twins will yield some answers about this in the near future.

53. How has biologic genetic research on schizophrenia been conducted in the past?

Before the late 1980s the biological research that was pursued on the genetics of schizophrenia was largely conducted by examining factors in blood, urine, and cerebral spinal fluid that were different in chronic patients with schizophrenia compared with controls. These numerous studies produced nothing consistent, and in fact many of those early positive findings were eventually found to be due to either the medications the patients were taking, their dietary differences, or the effects of institutionalization. When the field of molecular genetics began to explode in the early 1980s by producing multiple highly variable markers spread throughout the genome for specific genes, it became clear that these markers could be used to map the chromosomal location of different diseases and then be able, by identifying genes in the specific mapped location, to find a variation in a gene that leads to that specific disease. These methods then began to be applied to psychiatric disorders with genetic suscepti- bility, particularly schizophrenia.

54. What does linkage to a chromosome mean?

Many research groups worldwide began to evaluate families that by virtue of having more than one sibling with schizophrenia were considered ideal for these chromosomal **linkage** studies. The principles of genetic linkage studies are as follows: Our genes are organized in predetermined locations on pairs of 23 **chromosomes** (46 total). One of each pair is inherited from each parent. During reproduction, however, an independent assortment of the maternal and paternal genes on chromosome pairs exists so that the farther away genes are on each chromosome, the more the likelihood that different combinations of genes are inherited on the final chromosomes of the offspring of a mother–father pair. This is why no two siblings look alike unless they are identical twins and come from the same egg and sperm during fertilization. If there are known highly variable markers that could be spaced out across all chromosomes, one could then see which variations in the markers are present in each individual and trace the inheritance of variations in these markers down generations in families (Figure 1). In each fam-

Linkage

a genetic term that signifies a relation- ship between two or more genes on the same chromosome that are relatively close together so that sometimes the varia- tions in the traits that each represents are inherited together in the same individual.

Chromosome

a structure present in the nucleus of every cell of the body of any living thing con- taining genes. It is shaped like a long cylinder separated into two arms that are held together in the approximate middle by a structure called the cen- tromere.

ily, different variations in the markers will be present (because the mother has two and the father has two), but it is the position of the markers on chromosomes that is important, not the exact variation in the marker. Think of maps of towns. We have street names that vary and are different. The unique names help us locate houses on the streets. We can find the house because it is located between two named street signs. So it is with a disease gene. It is not the marker itself that will cause an illness, but it is the gene for an illness that is close to a specific marker that is important. If an illness gene is close to that marker, it will tend to be transmitted with the marker down generations, and we then say it is "linked." It is said to be "mapped" near that marker. **Geneticists**, based on this information in families with multiple ill and well members, are able to calculate how likely it is that a gene for illness is linked to a marker, given the pattern of marker inheritance that is observed in families such as the one illustrated in Figure 1. This method has been highly successful in the search to find genes for disorders known to be genetic, such as Huntington's chorea or phenylketonuria. A gene, however, such as one for schizophrenia, that may be only one of many that causes the same illness and that may have a non-traditional more complex mode of inheritance is not so easy to find by this method. In fact, the irony is that over the past decade there have been reports of many positive linkage findings for schizophrenia spread throughout all 23 chromosomes, and it has been difficult for researchers to tell which of these positives are true findings and which are falsely positive having been only chance findings. The key to this dilemma will be to find strong gene candidates whose involvement makes sense given their known functions and to corroborate these findings by other sources of evidence.

Geneticists

scientists who study the inheritance of traits in humans, animals, or plants.

CHROMOSOME 1 and its variants in markers. Only one of these variations is on a chromosome

___A,B,C,D,E,F_____G,H,I,J, K__SZ_____M,N,O_____

     Marker 1   Marker 2   Marker 3

Typical family pedigree and the inheritance of marker 2:

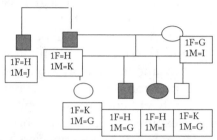

Figure 1. Illustration of linkage of schizophrenia to a chromosome if marker 2 on chromosome 1 is linked to schizophrenia (SZ). The boxes indicate the variants each person inherited. "F" is from the person's father and "M" is from the person's mother. ■ or ● = has schizophrenia ○ or □ = well. Circles are women and squares are males. Note that the "H" variant of marker 2 is present in all people who are ill in this family.

55. What are microarrays?

One of the other sources for genetic studies could be **microarray** experiments. To describe the new microarray technology, one first needs to mention that of all the genetic material in the human genome, only a very small amount of the DNA sequence actually leads to the production of proteins that, in turn, have a function in the body. The DNA that will be expressed is transferred into complementary sequences of messenger RNA (mRNA) that produce proteins critical to directing all bodily functions. This process is called gene expression. The process is complicated by many control mechanisms that enable the crucial timing of expression of genes and their turning on and off at different times in the life span of individuals. Microarrays are a new direct way to look at gene expression. Microarray technology enables researchers to examine the expression of thousands of genes at once in the

Microarray

this is an orderly arrangement of DNA samples to identify many genes at one time. They can contain thousands of genes on one small plate or "chip." An experiment with a single DNA chip or microarray can provide researchers information on thousands of genes simultaneously.

laboratory. The microarrays themselves are small slide or plate-like laboratory structures that support thousands of genes at fixed immobilized locations. The researcher places the genes in these locations in an orderly fashion, and thus, it is called an "array." If the expression of a gene is to be examined, the experiment is called "microarray expression analysis." If a gene is overexpressed in a certain disease state, then more of a sample of a sequence of expressed DNA will be present compared with control DNA. Arrays use fluorescent colors to quantify the amount of expression, and so if a particular gene expression is involved, it may be seen by expression of a different color. In schizophrenia research, microarray expression studies have been carried out on postmortem brains of patients who had chronic schizophrenia. Many results have come out of these studies, but it is still too early to tell whether the findings are consistent and relate to the findings from the linkage studies. Some early expression studies implicate genes for neuronal connectivity and growth. These studies, however, have so far not been able to clarify the effects that medication intake and other problems of illness chronicity and aging have on differential gene expression. In addition, examining brains of older people after death may not be useful for finding genes that are only expressed during brain development prenatally and in childhood.

56. What are the candidate genes for schizophrenia?

There have been claims from several linkage studies that genes within these regions that are known to be brain expressed could be involved in susceptibility for schizophrenia, but the exact nature of their roles has not been elucidated even in theories (Table 2). Aside from linkage and microarray studies, there are the so-called gene-association studies, where a specific variant in a gene is more frequent in populations of schizophrenic patients than in control populations. Many positive results have also come out of these studies because the standards for what consists of a positive finding have not yet been agreed on by researchers in the field. The following are the many genes that have been associated with schizophrenia by one method or another. What should be clear, however, is that no pathological defect has been found in any of these genes—that is, a mutation has not been found in people with schizophrenia and not in controls, with the possible exception of one or two reports in single rare families. These studies have not shown that within multiple families all those with schizophrenia have the putative variant, whereas those who do not have schizophrenia do not. The list of putative candidates includes brain-derived neurotrophic factor (BDNF), B-37, ciliary neurotrophic factor (CNTF), CNPase, COMT, DBH, DRD2, DRD3, DRD4, DISC I and DISC II, Dysbindin, 14-3-3-eta gene, G-72, G(olf), HSKCa3, HOPA, 5HT2a receptor, MAO-A and MAO-B, MAG, MAL, mGluR, MOG, neuregulin-1, nicotinic cholinergic receptor-α (CHRNA2), NOGO, NOTCH, PIP5K2A, PPP3CC (Calcineurin), proline oxidase, PRODH, RGS proteins, synapsin-III, synapsin-IIIa, TNF-α, tyrosine hydroxylase, and ZDHHC8. At the time of this writing, many, if not all, of these claimed genes could be false-positive research findings. Definitive replication studies are urgently needed.

Table 2. The Current Candidates in Linked Chromosomal Regions for Schizophrenia

Chromosome Location		Action
Disc I & II	1q	Unknown
Dysbindin	6p	Brain growth and development
Neuregulin-1	8p	Brain growth and development
PPP3CC Calcineurin	8p	Calmodulin dependent protein phosphatase
G72	13q	the Glutamate Pathway
COMT	22q	COMTDopamine metabolism
PRODH	22q	the Glutamate Pathway
ZDHHC8	22q	Palmitoylation
Synapsin IIIα	22q	Neuron connection plasticity
Protocadherin	X_2 and Y_p	Brain growth and development

57. How is it assumed that these genes cause schizophrenia?

Some general trends have been noticed about these genes, such as that some of them seem to converge on the neurochemical pathways for the nervous system nerve transmitter **glutamate**, whereas others are involved more specifically with functions involved in developing neuronal structural networks. These mechanisms are very interesting, but it is not yet known whether abnormalities in them have anything to do with why some people get schizophrenia.

58. What is an "intermediate phenotype" (sometimes called "endophenotype") for schizophrenia?

It is now thought that genes that cause schizophrenia likely act by affecting an "intermediate step"—that is, directly causing a change in the brain that will then in combination with other things lead to a vulnerability for developing schizophrenia, but that the genetic defects themselves will not be directly responsible for the illness as a whole (Figure 2). The most likely scenario is that one or more genes are defective in a certain way and that these genes are turned on and off during different stages of the lifespan of an individual, perhaps even in an abnormal timing mechanism as well. Thus, during prenatal development, some brain structures may develop abnormally in a subtle way; during adolescence, neuronal connections may abnormally form, and during aging, neurons may age in an accelerated or abnormal way. There will be less brain plasticity (Figure 3). All this is caused by abnormalities in the structure of one or more genes and/or its expression at different times during life.

**Glutaimine/
Glutamate**

an amino acid that is a building block of proteins. It is also by itself a major neurotransmitter in the brain (i.e., transmits information from cell to cell); by stimulating the activity of the cells, it excites them into activity.

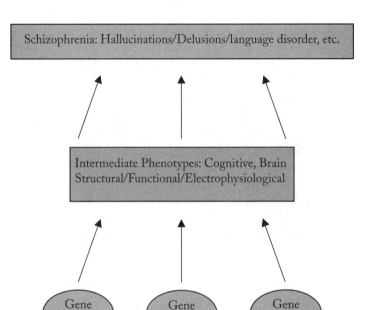

Figure 2.

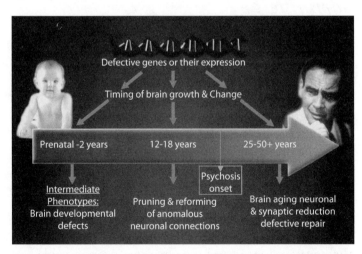

Figure 3. The concept that schizophrenia is a lifetime disorder with different genetically controlled events occuring at each stage by activation and deactivation of the same defective genes.

59. Will there be DNA testing for schizophrenia in the future?

It is highly unlikely that a specific genetic defect will be helpful for testing people to see whether they have inherited the tendency for schizophrenia. This is because, given the highly nonspecific biological and clinical findings in schizophrenia, no test will be likely to have enough sensitivity and specificity to be useful on a population basis for accurate testing. After genes are established that contribute to vulnerability, it is likely that their use will be confined to a scientific understanding of the mechanism for schizophrenia, which can then lead to the development of new medications.

60. Will DNA testing be useful in determining which medication to administer?

This could be another eventual use of DNA sequence variation among individuals. Although variation in specific gene DNA may not be associated with the illness itself, the medications that suppress its symptoms may be responded to in different ways depending on the genetic makeup of each individual. For example, if some people have **enzymes** that have higher activity for inactivating a certain medication, then these people may need higher doses to get a clinical response than people with lower enzyme activity will need, or these simply may not be responders to that particular medication. Similarly, if other individuals have low activity of an inactivating enzyme, they may have the drug in their system longer and thus be more prone to side effects. These factors, once established, could be available to clinicians so that they can tailor treatment with the many available drugs to each individual's unique genetic makeup. These principles belong to the new burgeoning field of "pharmacogenetics" and hold promise for the future but will need several years to develop and be useful.

Enzymes
proteins in the body that digest other substances through biochemical reactions. They are the "tools" of metabolism.

61. Can genetic research provide new treatments?

As stated previously here, an understanding of the biology of schizophrenia can only lead to better treatments, ones that can be given earlier, before pronounced clinical symptoms appear. Consumers, however, need to be aware that this is still a long time off. It takes many years for pharmaceutical companies to develop and test new drugs, and for every compound that the companies explore, many are abandoned for various reasons before they ever reach the market.

62. What are ethical concerns in this new genome age for the future?

Scientists must always take social responsibility for their new discoveries. Some families are happy to know that schizophrenia has a strong genetic component because then they know that it has been out of their control and that their behavior was not responsible for making someone ill in their family. Other families, in contrast, see that they have somehow been stigmatized and are passing on "bad blood." Scientists in collaboration with lawmakers must develop legislation that prevents the misuses of genetic data to label individuals as unfit so that these individuals will not be prevented from obtaining health insurance policies and educational and employment opportunities available to others in society. There is also the concern that people will want genetic testing before mating so as not to raise a child who is likely to get this illness or will think twice about marrying someone with a family history of this illness, despite scientific knowledge that the excess genetic risk is low and not understood. You could envision numerous scenarios coming from superficial knowledge that schizophrenia is genetic.

Part Five

The Biology Underlying Schizophrenia: Current Research Findings

"I think you have to speculate. If I have a good idea, I tend to believe it is true. An idea is better than no idea ... that's the way good science works. An idea can be tested, whereas if you have no idea, nothing can be tested and you don't understand anything!"

James D. Watson in an interview published in *NY Times*,
On the 50th Anniversary of the Discovery of DNA
February 3, 2002

63. Are there any tests that can be taken from blood, urine, or spinal fluid?

The answer is none at all, unlike most other biologic disease. You can find high blood sugar in diabetes or elevated **immunoglobulins** in multiple sclerosis. If only we had a good hypothesis about what to look for in schizophrenia! For years, factors were found in 24-hour urine collections, serum, and spinal fluid. The notorious "pink spot," a supposed litmus test for schizophrenia, was none other than metabolites of tea that the patients were drinking in excess. The so-called endogenous hallucinogens, chemicals produced in excess by one's own body, such as dimethyltryptamine and phenylethylamine, both turned out also to be artifactual findings, the former being caused by a laboratory method that had not been validated and the latter caused by nonspecific anxiety.

64. Are there any differences in the brains of people that have schizophrenia?

Yes, but in a subtle way, and no finding is specific to the illness nor is any one finding present in all patients with schizophrenia. Someone with schizophrenia could also have a completely normal brain. Since the beginning of the recognition of the concept of "Dementia Praecox," Kraepelin (1907) felt that this was a progressive brain disease, and he noted in his textbook that "the course is progressive without remissions…. Signs of mental deterioration may appear within a few months, and are usually well marked by the end of two years….On the other hand, there are some cases … which do not dement for a number of years." He also said early on (Kraepelin, 1899) that "in view of the clinical and anatomical facts known so far I cannot doubt we are dealing with serious … and only partially reversible damage to the cerebral **cortex**…. 75 percent of cases reach higher grades of dementia and sink deeper and deeper." By the time he published his 1919 text, he illustrated what he thought was wrong in

Immunoglobulins

the proteins that help the body respond to foreign substances and infections.

Cortex (cerebral cortex)

the outer portion of the brain. It consists mostly of the "gray matter" that contains nerve cells.

the brain with drawings of neurons that he described as "diseased with lipoid products of disintegration." Where his notions about the brain came from, however, are unclear, as there are no careful research studies that he or anyone else published to provide evidence of these claims.

By the 1930s the technique of examining the brain by **pneumoencephalography**, a quite risky procedure of injecting air into the **ventricles** (the space that holds the cerebral spinal fluid that bathes the brain) in order to observe their outline, was applied to studies of patients with schizophrenia. Many reports showed enlargement of the ventricular space in chronic schizophrenia, clearly suggestive of atrophy of the brain at an age when this should not have been present. These results went quite unnoticed by most psychiatrists in the mid 20th century, probably because of the rise in psychological and psychoanalytic theories and approaches to schizophrenia. When biological psychiatry again became in vogue and new methods to examine the brain *in vivo* were developed, namely **computed tomography** (CT), some exciting findings emerged. In 1976 a very small study of severely ill patients with chronic schizophrenia was published in the medical journal *The Lancet* (Johnstone et al., 1976). It clearly showed by CT that the patients had significantly larger brain ventricular size than age-matched controls. Soon many other investigators, using much larger, more representative samples of patients, widely replicated this finding. To date, this is probably the most replicated finding in all of schizophrenia research! In the late 1980s brain-imaging methods produced even better direct anatomical windows into the *in vivo* brain with the advent of **magnetic resonance imaging** (MRI) scanners. The first studies, however, were performed using brain slices that were very thick so subtle changes that occur in small brain structures or just subtle differences in general could be easily missed. Over the decade that followed, however, MRI scanning became more and

Pneumoencephalography

an X-ray picture of the brain taken by injection of air into the cerebral ventricular space.

Ventricles

as this term applies to the brain, the spaces connecting throughout the brain that provide a system for the circulation of the fluid present in the brain called cerebrospinal fluid.

Computed tomography (CT)

a form of X-ray that is able to view the brain in more detail than a standard skull X-ray.

Magnetic resonance imaging

a method to examine the tissue of the brain using a magnetic field and computer system.

Gray matter

the brownish-gray nerve tissue of the brain and spinal cord that contains the nerve cells.

White matter

whitish brain and spinal cord tissue composed mostly of nerve fibers and its shiny protective coat called myelin.

Superior temporal gyrus

a portion of the temporal lobe of the brain that has many functions related to language, including hearing it and speaking it.

more refined and brain images came to be seen in almost as much detail and contrast as direct post-mortem brain visualization. MRI scanning currently is the main imaging technique used to evaluate the brains of people with schizophrenia. In MRI the actual brain tissue, divided into the **gray matter** containing the neuronal cells and the **white matter** containing their fibrous connections, is clearly distinguishable. As a result, a number of studies have shown various differences in the brains of patients with schizophrenia. These mostly include volume of structures. Besides the ventricles, the volume of gray matter as a whole is significantly less, as is the size of the temporal lobe and its different subdivisions (i.e., **superior temporal gyrus** and hippocampus), frontal lobe, and corpus callosum (Table 3) (Figure 4).

We now know that there are also white matter changes in these structures.

Table 3.

Brain Structure	Ventricles	Frontal Lobes	Temporal Lobes Superior Temporal Gyrus Hippocampus
Structure Function	Holds spinal fluid that bathes the brain	Sequential planning Processing new memory Speaking Some uniquely human mentalizing	Language memory
Finding in some people with schizophrenia	Enlarged	Reduced volume in parts.	Reduced volume in parts.
Does the finding progress over time?	Yes	Unknown	Possibly for all
Comments	Large ventricles mean that the brain tissue surrounding it is less than it should be.	This structure is difficult to measure, but its functioning has been shown in many ways to be abnormal.	

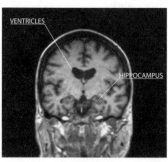 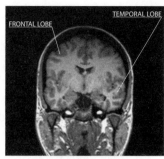

Figure 4. (1) MRI -- Patient with schizophrenia. (2) MRI -- Normal person.

65. Should an MRI scan be performed?

In a clinical setting, a good evaluation of someone who is first being diagnosed with schizophrenia should include an MRI so that a baseline initial brain assessment is available for comparison in later years. It should also be used to exclude any other brain diseases that could mimic the symptoms of schizophrenia, such as temporal lobe tumors, or any other known neurodegenerative disorder, no matter how rare they are in people with characteristic symptoms of schizophrenia. The status of brain structural and functional findings could be helpful for considering what the likely outcome of an episode might be.

66. Are functional MRI scans useful?

Some other types of MRI scans that can be performed are **functional MRI** (fMRI) or **magnetic resonance spectroscopy** (MRS). In fMRI, subjects are given a test to perform that uses different brain anatomical regions while the scanner takes pictures of their brain. In patients with schizophrenia, the tasks usually include some type of behavior that requires a short period of memory or language detection by responding when hearing instructions or when seeing them. In general, the functioning of different parts of the brain is measurable by the intensity of activity in the working regions. Schizophrenia patients have been shown

Functional MRI

a brain scan that shows actions taking place in the brain in response to a stimulus. The stimulus could be anything, such as voluntary movement of the fingers to memorizing a set of words.

Magnetic resonance spectroscopy

a type of MRI scan that examines chemical spectras in the brain. These chemicals are those that are present in the structure of membranes or metabolic activity in nerve cells and between cells.

to have less focused and less lateralized functioning when responding to these tasks, although these studies are just initial research findings. More needs to be done before this kind of scanning can be applied in clinical situations. Similarly, MRS is a quantitative imaging method to detect levels of metabolized neuro-chemicals in the brain in different regions. Abnormal amounts of these substances are thought to indicate evidence of progressive brain disease at the biochemical level. These scans too, however, are not applicable to a clinical setting and have only been research tools that present some complicated problems thus far in their interpretation.

67. Should an EEG be done on patients with schizophrenia?

Certain findings in EEG scans are characteristic of people with schizophrenia. For example, some of the EEG brain waves that are produced when the subject is stimulated in some way are known as "evoked potentials." Patients with schizophrenia have reduced amplitudes of these waves, particularly over the frontal and temporal lobes, when they are stimulated with an odd sound or visual object. These tests might also be worth conducting because they are associated with other symptoms and similar to the MRI might be able to give some prognostic indication. However, for the most part, they are still considered research tools and not available in a clinical setting.

68. Is schizophrenia a "chemical imbalance"?

Many people speak of schizophrenia as a "chemical imbalance," which makes sense given that the medications are chemicals that alleviate many symptoms. What this actually means, however, is still not clear in research studies, and how the chemistry interacts with the structural brain changes is not known. Many biochemical hypotheses about schizophrenia were espoused after neuroleptic medications were introduced. These drugs act directly on **dopamine** receptors, as well as other receptors, and their efficacy could be shown to be directly related specifically to dopamine activity by laboratory assays. Consequently, the dopamine hypothesis has always been the most prominent. In support of the dopamine hypothesis are studies showing that dopamine receptors measured in postmortem brain and also in **positron emission tomography** (PET) scans were elevated in patients with schizophrenia. Some evidence showed that these findings were not due to an effect of the medication, but rather the pathology of the illness itself. **Serotonin**, another brain neurotransmitter, as well as GABA and others, has been thought to be related somehow to schizophrenia pathology and likely by their effects on dopamine receptors.

More recently, the "glutamate hypothesis" has become even more prominent than the dopamine hypothesis. L-Glutamic acid (glutamate) is a major excitatory amino acid neurotransmitter throughout the brain and nervous system, and it is known that glutamate plays a major role in brain development, affecting neuronal migration, neuronal differentiation, axon genesis, and neuronal survival. It first was thought to be involved in schizophrenia; the popular recreational drug phencyclidine (PCP) was recognized to not only mimic schizophrenia in its actions, but also to exert its actions primarily on glutamate receptors. Several lines of evidence then suggested that a dysfunction in glutamatergic neurotransmission via the N-methyl-d-aspartate (NMDA) subtype of glutamate receptors might be involved in the pathophysiology of schizophrenia, and the NMDA receptor hypofunction hypothesis of schizophrenia became known. The dopamine hypothesis attributes hyperdopaminergic function as a possible cause of schizophrenia, whereas the glutamate hypothesis proposes a hypofunctional glutamate system. There is substantial evidence for

Dopamine

a chemical substance that is important for conveying "messages" between nerve cells in the brain.

Positron emission tomography (PET Scanning)

this is a radiologic procedure that measures the metabolism of a radiolabeled substance that is injected into a subject's vein and one that is known to enter the brain relatively rapidly.

Serotonin

a hormone found in the brain, platelets, digestive tract, and pineal gland. It acts both as a neurotransmitter (a substance that nerves use to send messages to one another) and a vasoconstrictor (a substance that causes blood vessels to narrow). A lack of serotonin in the brain is thought to be a cause of depression.

both hypotheses, based on observations that certain classes of street drugs can produce schizophrenic-like symptoms in normal individuals. Not only does PCP produce symptoms most similar to schizophrenia by antagonizing the action of glutamate, but amphetamines also produce some of the acute positive symptoms by stimulating dopamine receptors. In general, PCP and similar drugs produce somewhat more of the positive and negative symptoms of schizophrenia than the amphetamine-like drugs. The latter fail to produce some of the core symptoms of schizophrenia, such as formal thought disorder and negative symptoms, although PCP may. Currently, initiated by the glutamate hypothesis, both glycine and d-serine, NMDA receptor stimulators, are being used as add-on medications to treat patients with chronic schizophrenia who do not completely benefit from other medications.

69. When do these brain changes occur, and is schizophrenia considered a progressive brain disorder?

Patients with chronic schizophrenia are known to have the changes mentioned previously that are recognized in brain structures, but when they begin to become abnormal in the lifetime of an individual is still controversial. Studies of patients at the first episode, however, are able to detect many of the changes, suggesting that they may occur early. There is some evidence from a couple of recent high-risk studies that the brain changes actually predate illness and the brain continues to deteriorate along with the development of symptoms. More research is needed on this topic, but its implications are vast. If there is progressive brain structural change characteristic of schizophrenia and it is related to the evolution of clinical symptoms, then medications need to be given early to prevent progression. Several research groups are now working on this issue and hopefully will soon produce recommendations about early treatment and the types of treatment.

70. What is the neurodevelopmental hypothesis about schizophrenia?

For over a decade most investigators have thought that the brain structural abnormalities of schizophrenia must at least in part be neurodevelopmental in origin—that is, occurring either because of an insult prenatally to the developing brain or because of a neuronal growth defect prenatally that is perhaps genetically controlled. One alternative hypothesis was that in adolescent-onset illness, the reorganization of brain connections during that time might be occurring abnormally. The reasons for constructing these theories as an alternative to thinking of schizophrenia as a progressive degenerative process mainly were that the length of illness duration could never be correlated with the amount of abnormal brain change and that no cellular signs of degeneration have ever been shown in brains of patients with schizophrenia. It has now become clear, however, from results of carefully conducted longitudinal studies that brain ventricular size continues to expand over time and that none of the anomalies associated with schizophrenia appear static. See Figure 3 in part four on "Genetic Risk" for a combination of both the neurodevelopmental and degenerative hypotheses. Table 3 in this chapter outlines the changes that have been found in brains of patients with schizophrenia and whether there is evidence of progressive change in these structures. Figure 5 illustrates an example of one such case of a young 34-year-old female with schizophrenia whose ventricles appear to have consistently enlarged over time from her first episode of illness to 5 and then 10 years later.

Figure 5. 10-year MRI follow-up. 34-year-old female with chronic schizophrenia and a brother with schizophrenia as well.

R			L
Feb. 1990	Feb. 1995	Jan. 2000	
1st Episode	5 years later	10 years later	

Part Six

Substance Abuse and Schizophrenia

"It was very well to say 'Drink me,'" but the wise little Alice was not going to do that in a hurry. 'No, I'll look first,' she said, 'and see whether it is marked "poison" or not.' . . . However, this bottle was not marked 'poison,' so Alice ventured to taste it, and finding it very nice . . . very soon finished it off."

Down the Rabbit-Hole, *Alice's Adventures in Wonderland*, by Lewis Carroll, 1865

71. Can drug use in adolescence cause schizophrenia?

It has long been known that various street drugs are used by people who develop an acute first episode of schizophrenia and that patients and their families often blame the first episode on these drugs. Although there is an increased drug use in people developing schizophrenia compared with those who do not of similar ages, it has long been controversial as to which really comes first, drug abuse or schizophrenia. Can certain drugs cause schizophrenia, or does having subtle emotional signs of "preschizophrenia" cause people to alleviate their uncomfortable feelings or behaviors by experimenting with drugs? Some data from Europe recently indicate that in some people who are frequent drug users, particularly of cannabis (marijuana), the use of drugs may be causal. However, it is generally thought that because many people who use cannabis or other drugs frequently do *not* get schizophrenia, a genetic predisposition to get the illness must also be present. Alternatively, the use of drugs may simply bring what is already a predetermined illness on faster. Drug use has been associated with an earlier age of onset of schizophrenia and with a poorer outcome and is particularly relevant to males with the illness, as males tend to abuse drugs significantly more than females. The kind of drug that can be harmful also differs across the world and depends on what is popular during a particular era and what is readily available. This, of course, varies geographically and with time. Various drugs that have been used and were popular at different points in time were also known by various street names but include amphetamines (speed or ecstasy), PCP, lysergic acid diethylamide (LSD), cannabis (hash, marijuana). LSD was the drug of the 1960s to the point that songs were popularized about its use (e.g., "Lucy in the Sky with Diamonds"). Particularly LSD and PCP are considered hallucinogens in normal individuals, although others have been used as such at different times, whereas cannabis in normal individuals is not considered hallucinogenic, despite its association with schizophrenia.

72. Can someone who has schizophrenia smoke marijuana?

Numerous studies now show a strong association between marijuana use and the development of schizophrenia. Thus, it would not be advisable for people already diagnosed with schizophrenia to use marijuana. Some believe that this newly reported association results from an increased potency in the marijuana now available on the streets, which has increased substantially over recent years. After schizophrenia is diagnosed, continued use of cannabis or marijuana, easily available compared with other street drugs, can only be harmful in causing less likelihood of response to medication. It also initiates a lack of compliance with oral medication by the patients so that they tend to have a poor outcome and become rehospitalized until they realize the need to stay away from it. Their reactions are often not euphoric and calming as the effects on their peers who do not have schizophrenia, although the mechanism for this difference is not known.

73. Are there any specific drugs that more frequently cause schizophrenia-like symptoms?

No street drugs are free from this association. Some of them, such as methamphetamines and PCP, are known to mimic symptoms of schizophrenia acutely in otherwise normal people who are given doses of them. Both of these drugs are epidemic in some countries. Methamphetamine use is particularly high and widely prevalent in many African countries, and thus psychiatrists in these countries are finding difficulty separating true chronic schizophrenia from continuous methamphetamine use.

74. Is it okay to drink alcohol if you have schizophrenia?

The simple answer is no. Alcohol, particularly in moderate amounts, only precipitates both affective symptoms and exacerbates the symptoms of schizophrenia as well as leads to noncompliance with a medication regime and rehospitalization in many people. It is certainly not advised, given that it is not easily used in careful moderation. One beer at night on a social occasion for someone with schizophrenia may even be beneficial if it affords a way of socializing and meeting with peers—that is, becoming more integrated into everyday life. It is the excess that is harmful to anyone, and those with schizophrenia are particularly sensitive.

75. Why do people with schizophrenia smoke cigarettes excessively?

It has long been noticed that patients on psychiatric hospital wards are almost all chain cigarette smokers, and numerous scientific surveys now confirm the association of cigarette smoking with schizophrenia. Behavioral therapies in the past were geared toward positive reinforcement by the attainment of a goal and thus winning a pack of cigarettes. You might think that the consequence of this would be that lung cancer and other cigarette-associated cancers would also be increased in schizophrenic patients, but this does not appear to be true. Whether people with schizophrenia smoke cigarettes because of their underlying psychopathology or because of a social consequence of having this illness is presently unclear. It may simply be that these people develop the addictive habit of cigarette smoking because of a need to occupy their hands and stimulate themselves with some oral gratification during times that are continually stressful and uncomfortable. This phenomenon was recently noted to have a specific scientific basis by a well-known researcher in Colorado, Dr. Robert Freedman, who claims that cigarette smoking is so excessive among these patients, namely a craving for nicotine, because of an underlying abnormality in receptors for nicotine in the brain. His laboratory is currently studying nicotine receptors in people with schizophrenia, the genetic susceptibility for abnormalities in these receptors, and possible medications that can counteract the abnormal effects. None, however, has been found to date to be effective in alleviating the symptoms of schizophrenia.

Part Seven

Violence and Aggression in Schizophrenia

"Is this a dagger I see before me,
The handle toward my hand? Come, let me clutch thee,....
I go, and it is done. The bell invites me.
Hear it not, Duncan; for it is a knell
That summons thee to heaven or to hell."

Shakespeare, *Macbeth*, Act 2, Scene 1

76. Do people with schizophrenia frequently commit violent acts?

Violence is *not* a symptom of schizophrenia. An individual with schizophrenia is not more dangerous than any other person, provided that he or she is treated with medication for symptoms. In fact, people with schizophrenia are far more likely to harm themselves than others. However, there is a conception that people with schizophrenia are violent. This notion is likely to be based particularly on cases that gain a lot of publicity and are subjects of movies, such as the paranoid schizophrenia patient who was released from a Long Island, New York, state psychiatric hospital, convincing his physician that he no longer had the delusion that his estranged wife must die, only to immediately go to her home and murder her, or the homeless hallucinating man who pushed a young girl onto the New York City subway track and into the path of an incoming train. Ted Kaczynski, the "Unabomber," was clearly suffering from paranoid schizophrenia and a thought disorder that was certainly evident in the manifesto he sent to *The New York Times.* In the United Kingdom, a serial killer known as the "Yorkshire Ripper," suffered from schizophrenia and was committed to a long-stay psychiatric forensic hospital after his trial. The young man with severe paranoia who shot many random people on the Long Island Railroad certainly had all the signs of untreated paranoid schizophrenia for years, but most people did not pay enough attention to getting him to treatment. Finally, the famous young man John Hinckley, Jr., who felt the delusional need to shoot President Reagan many years ago, was diagnosed with schizophrenia and has spent many years since in a psychiatric hospital. This particular case, similar to the Long Island Railroad shooter, was one in which the affected individual had a long history of unstable behavior and several warning signs of psychopathological behavior that should have led family, friends, and professionals to intervene much earlier. He became over the years obsessed with the movie *Taxi Driver*, which was about an American psychopath who stalks the president of the United States. The actress, Jodie Foster, played an attractive young woman in the movie, who John saw himself becoming romantically involved with to the point of stalking her with letters and attempted visits while she was a student at Yale. Some people say that his obsession with this movie is what drove him to purchase handguns and eventually on March 29, 1981, to shoot and wound President Reagan and his press secretary James Brady, as well as two other individuals on the scene. He was tried and eventually found not guilty by reason of insanity and sent to the special forensic unit at St. Elizabeth's Hospital in Washington, DC. The tragedy is that if any of the professionals, including psychiatrists, who he had seen during the several years preceding this event had identified the correct diagnosis and treated him with neuroleptic medication, the violence he inflicted on the president and others would likely not have occurred. Many such stories give the public the impression that people with schizophrenia, by virtue of their diagnosis, are dangerous. Despite some of the previous examples, when violence does occur, it is most frequently targeted at family members and is not premeditated. In addition, all these examples of violent crimes were committed when the perpetrator was in an unstable stage of illness that was untreated. The subway incident described previously here was the stimulus for New York State to pass a mandatory outpatient treatment law (Kendra's Law, named after the girl who was pushed onto the subway tracks and died) so that patients with schizophrenia who are released from hospitals cannot voluntarily choose to discontinue their medications.

77. Is there research on how violent behavior can be predicted?

The likelihood of violence is increased by alcohol or street drug intake and noncompliance with the pre-

scribed medication regime. The most important predictor of violent behavior is a past history of violence,
whether or not someone has schizophrenia. Strong
predictors of violence in the mentally ill are the feeling
that others are out to harm one's self and the feeling
that one's mind is dominated by forces beyond self-
control or that thoughts are being put into one's head.
Another symptom that may predict violence is a specific type of hallucination called "command hallucinations," in which internal voices are heard as if they
were coming from the outside telling the individual
what to do and in many cases to either harm one's self
or someone else. The presence of this type of hallucination and the need to act on it may be a compelling
predictor of violence. Of course, the strongest predictor of violence is having performed violent acts in the
past.

Often, however, police pick up individuals with schizophrenia as a precautionary measure because they do
not know when someone who is behaving out of the
ordinary is likely to be violent. Such is especially true
in Washington, DC, where caution may be essential
but can sometimes be an overreaction. For example, it
is common for many people with paranoid or other
types of schizophrenia from all over the country to
travel to the nation's capital to address their many
delusions about the FBI, the Internal Revenue Service,
or even the president. At St. Elizabeth's Hospital, the
once only Federal Psychiatric Institution, in the late
20th century and for many years, a special ward existed
in the forensic division for the "White House cases."
Anyone who threatened the president would be
brought there and could not be released until the
Secret Service allowed it. On one occasion I evaluated
a patient on this ward whose only crime was feeling
that he had many things in common with the then-
president Gerald Ford and simply presented himself at
the gate of the White House requesting to "share his
bubble gum with President Ford!" Education of law
enforcement officers, the Secret Service, and the FBI

in how to predict violent behavior and also manage patients with schizophrenia is essential.

78. Do people with schizophrenia more frequently commit crimes?

Crimes are not only acts of violence. Various other crimes, such as robbery, property damage, and many infractions of the law, can lead to jail sentences. Antisocial behavior, commonly known as psychopathy, is clearly associated with crime. Large studies of individuals with and without schizophrenia, however, do not suggest that psychopathy is associated with schizophrenia; regardless of psychotic diagnosis, it is associated with crime. In addition, family studies do not show an excess clustering of psychopathy among relatives of schizophrenic patients, indicating that this behavior is not genetically associated with schizophrenia.

79. What should I do if my relative or friend is behaving violently?

Many people close to patients with schizophrenia are frustrated with the mental health care system as it currently exists in the United States because in most instances it does not provide support for a sick individual until he or she is behaving dangerously toward others or acutely threatening suicide. In these circumstances, of course, the police emergency phone number should be called immediately, and the patient must be subdued and brought to a psychiatric hospital. Unfortunately, these patients are too often victims of accidental violence by frightened police who then provide severe force to suppress the violent individuals and in some cases inflict injuries and even death. Police forces and all types of public emergency response personnel must be trained in the acute care of these individuals and how to safely transport them to psychiatric emergency rooms. Too often, patients are instead brought to jail and kept there for many days without much-needed medications. Families and friends can be instrumental support at times like these to ensure that patients receive the proper treatment and legal representation.

Part Eight

Suicidal Behavior and Schizophrenia

"They heard her singing her last song,
The Lady of Shalott ....
Till her blood was frozen slowly,
And her eyes were darkened wholly. ...
Who is this? And what is here?
And in the lighted palace near
Died the sound of royal cheer ...
But Lancelot mused a little space;
He said, "She has a lovely face;
God in his mercy lend her grace,
The Lady of Shalott."

Alfred Lord Tennyson, "The Lady of Shalott," Part IV

80. What are the signs of suicidal thoughts in schizophrenia?

It is commonly thought that suicide is solely a characteristic of depression, but this is not so. Approximately 1 in 10 people with schizophrenia commit suicide, and thus the average age span of people with schizophrenia is less than that of the general population. Suicide attempts are even several fold more common than the cases that are successfully completed. The most vulnerable period for suicide is when most people with this diagnosis are young, newly diagnosed, treated with medications for the first time, and then recently discharged from the hospital. Often these individuals have not been connected properly to supportive networks and regular treatment. They have also not been adequately educated about their illness and the need for continual medication. Frequently, they are in a state of denial so that after the symptoms have subsided, they will be back to their premorbid state and will discontinue any medication recommended. However, they find adjustment to their old lives and being able to return to the independence that they enjoyed difficult. Many friends have deserted them, and a general lack of connection and closeness exists to other people as a result. This is a period when strong support, guidance, and frequent professional observation and follow-up are needed. In addition, not being married, coming from a high socioeconomic family background, and having high intelligence and high life expectations all lead to a feeling of loss, hopelessness, and isolation. If the individual then does not comply with the prescribed treatments and turns to street drugs, the suicidal risk increases substantially. With regard to symptoms that are likely to lead to suicide, depression, of course, is by far the most common among individuals with schizophrenia, as it is in all cases of suicide. Less frequently present are the paranoid attacks of panic that lead to suicidal acts and provide the only way out of the delusion of being chased or followed. Occasionally, patients are responding to voices commanding them to harm themselves. In contrast to public understanding, depression is present in the majority of people with schizophrenia at some time during the course of their illness.

In the book *Night Falls Fast*, Kay Jamison describes the development of psychotic and depressive behavior in a close friend that eventually led to suicide. Could this have been prevented if she had been there for him? This was one of the reflections that she will never be able to answer. The book, however, clearly describes all the signs of impending suicide and how one may survive them, as she herself did. Similarly, the Foreword to this book illustrates one family's struggle with a young loved one who eventually committed suicide because of the "pain." Thus, the subtitle of this book is "Painful Minds."

81. What can be done to prevent suicide attempts?

The foremost important prevention measure is to provide intensive frequent follow-up for newly diagnosed patients. Support systems must be in place before release of such patients from the hospital, and these must include not only psychiatric care but also occupational rehabilitation, family support, social support, financial support, and then finally, follow-up of healthcare personnel to make sure that a comprehensive treatment plan occurs. It is now thought that certain medications may be particularly beneficial and protective against suicidal thoughts, although the mechanism for this action is not clearly understood. One such medication that has been shown in a large trial to lead to significantly less suicidal behavior than other medications is clozapine. This effect may be due to clozapine's prominent stimulant action on serotonin receptors in the brain, although this is only a theory. Suicide has long been associated with low brain levels of the metabolites of serotonin and may indicate low serotonergic tone in the brain. Serotonin is a neurotransmitter that is abundant in brain regions that are associated with emotion. It is thus possible that low moods are a reflection of low serotonin, which is supported by the knowledge that newer antidepressants called the serotonin receptor uptake inhibitors (SSRIs) raise the availability of serotonin in brain tissue and are helpful in alleviating depression.

Part Nine

Issues for Women

"The day will come when men will recognize woman as his peer, not only at the fireside, but in councils of the nation. Then, and not until then, will there be a perfect comradeship, the ideal union between the sexes that will result in the highest development of the race."

Susan B. Anthony

"Remember, no one can make you feel inferior without your consent."

Eleanor Roosevelt

"Tell us what it is to be a woman so that we may know what it is to be a man."

Toni Morrison, Nobel Lecture, 1993

82. Is schizophrenia different in women?

For many years in the United States and elsewhere, women were placed in psychiatric hospitals for long periods of time and institutionalized simply for having a domineering husband and dysfunctional family life. Husbands who wished to discard their wives could sign commitment papers and claim psychiatric symptoms in their wives in order to do so. Geller and Harris (1994) have documented the histories of typical women of this sort from as early as 1840 through 1945. More humane treatment and legislation against involuntary hospitalization for less than acutely dangerous conditions have abolished these inequities, but they remain documented in the history of psychiatry. In fact, there is no reason to keep many women hospitalized for long periods of time, as schizophrenia has a much better outcome in women than men overall. Women have a later age of onset than men on average and may also have a different cluster of symptoms and are more likely to have a brief psychotic episode that resolves more quickly than men. Women also are less aggressive than men when unmedicated and thus not a danger to other people. The poorer social outcome for men than women can be attributed to having reached less of a level of social development by the time of onset than women. Thus, age at onset of the biology of schizophrenia may be the key variable. Late-onset schizophrenia (over the age of 40) is almost exclusively in women. The women are more often diagnosed with schizoaffective disorder and less likely with paranoid schizophrenia than men, but how much of this difference might be cultural, at least in part, is unknown. Pharmacotherapy in women should also be different because the response of women to medications may differ from men. They require lower doses in order to suppress symptoms, and some serious side effects are more often seen in women than men. Drug trials, however, specifically comparing women with men that are controlled for various environmental and other factors that could affect drug levels and thus treatment response (such as cigarette smoking), are far too few.

Women tend to be ignored and even eliminated from research clinical trials.

A common notion to explain sex differences is that **estrogen** levels must have a protective effect on the development of schizophrenia. Studies show a modulation of the dopamine D2 receptors by estrogen and also that estrogen in some studies has a weak neuroleptic-like effect. This is not the only explanation for sex differences, however. In fact, genetics also clearly plays a role in actual age of onset. Despite the age of onset for schizophrenia being on average a couple of years later in women than men, when more than one individual within a family has schizophrenia, the age of onset tends to be highly similar regardless of the sex of the affected individuals. This implies that inheritance also influences the age of onset. If the sex differences in schizophrenia are genetic, then a gene that at least modifies the illness expression, or even causes it entirely, may be on the sex chromosomes. Although this theory has not yet been proven, it is currently openly debated (DeLisi & Crow, 1989).

Estrogen
a female hormone that is produced in the female organs (ovaries). It is produced in different amounts throughout the menstrual cycle and is reduced after menopause.

83. Should patients who are pregnant take medication for schizophrenia?

Women who take antipsychotic medication, because of its hyperprolactin effects, are less fertile than women who are not on these medications. Exposing the developing infant prenatally or through lactation to antipsychotic medication could have long-term sequelae. The conventional neuroleptics do have an increased risk of congenital malformations, particularly during the earlier weeks of pregnancy (weeks 4 through 10). The establishment of recommended dosing for women during pregnancy, however, has not been adequately studied, nor has any treatment trial been performed comparing different neuroleptic treatments for their subsequent effect on the developing fetus. The lack of this research is unwarranted, but even to date, it goes unnoticed. The excuse of many researchers usually is that hormonal changes cannot be controlled in research studies, thus making interpretation of any study results on women difficult. It also may be, however, that the hormonal modification of the action of some neuroleptics may allow for lower doses to be given during pregnancy, but this needs to be carefully examined. The pharmacologic management of women in the perinatal period when hormonal status suddenly changes is also very important, and little has been described about this condition in the literature. Having schizophrenia also leads to an increased risk for obstetrical complications, including preterm deliveries and a low-birthweight infant. The interaction of obstetric complications with whether the mother is medicated with neuroleptics and psychiatrically stable is unknown. In general, women with schizophrenia also tend to receive poorer prenatal medical care, and this too may lead to complications as a consequence. It is clear that not enough research has been done on pregnancy in schizophrenia. Overall, the risk of withholding medication to suppress psychosis must be weighed against the risk to the fetus and to the mother.

In addition, women with schizophrenia have higher rates of forced sex and unwanted pregnancies. They may also have a reduced capacity to provide mothering and to respond to their child's needs and need special guidance to overcome and deal with these circumstances and deficits.

84. What is the risk of a postpartum relapse?

Special support after birth for women with schizophrenia needs to be intensive and postpartum relapse prevented or detected early so that treatment can quickly be augmented. The risk of a postpartum psychiatric disorder is higher in women with a prior psychiatric history than those without it, particularly depression and psychosis. The change in hormone levels during the perinatal period may also warrant change in neuroleptic dose. Unfortunately, there have been too many highly publicized cases in the United States of mothers who either have a postpartum relapse of their illness or have a first episode of a psychosis during the postpartum period as long as six months after giving birth. At the extreme, these women can be very harmful to their children and have been known to kill them because of various delusional beliefs, such as in the famous Andrea Yates case. Mrs. Yates had multiple delusions about her children being cursed by the devil, and she acted upon her need to supposedly end their suffering by drowning them one by one. Her husband was remarkably unaware that she had psychiatric problems and failed to pick up on any warning signs. Such tragic events could be avoided with careful recognition and treatment of high-risk postpartum women by healthcare professionals and the education of close family members.

85. What about breast-feeding?

Postpartum lactation and breast-feeding may augment the higher prolactin levels already present during conventional antipsychotic treatment. Breast milk, however, likely excretes neuroleptics and thus breast-feeding should be cautioned against in medicated patients. We do not know the effect of neuroleptics on the developing infant but assume that there could be lasting effects on the brain and nervous system. There are no studies of children of breast-feeding patients on neuroleptics, nor are there studies of the new atypical neuroleptics to see whether they are safer than old generation neuroleptics for women. It is presently unknown whether any of these medications, including antidepressants, affect brain growth and development. Thus, it is recommended that women on these medications do not breast-feed their children. It is hoped that the pharmaceutical industry will take the responsibility to investigate these important issues in the near future.

86. Does the concept "schizophrenogenic mother" exist?

In the 1960s the concept that schizophrenia was due to miscommunication among members of a nuclear family was a very popular concept. The mother, who had a more intense interaction with the child from infancy on, was considered to be the one who had the most influence and most chance to transmit miscommunications that were termed "schizophrenigenic." A famous analyst, Freida-Fromm Reichman, was known to espouse the theory of regressing patients back to infancy and then bringing the patient back to his or her current age with a particular kind of analysis that claimed to recreate the mothering that was never received. Unfortunately, this concept has caused much harm to families and their relationships with psychiatrists trying to treat the patient. Currently, no scientific basis suggests that a mother's communication style is harmful to a young child and can cause later schizophrenia.

87. Can estrogen for birth control help suppress symptoms?

Often women who have schizophrenia and are sexually active do not use contraceptives and frequently are not compliant with oral contraceptives; thus, if warranted, the use of long-acting contraceptive medications is the method of choice. Whether these treatments augment the effects of antipsychotic medication has been little studied. Although there have been studies to suggest this, as mentioned previously here, large-scale studies of women have not been a focus in research studies. It is also of interest that drug trials of the new antipsychotics that do include women do not standardize whether women are administered oral contraceptives. Again, systematic trials need to be supported by the pharmaceutical companies because a few small studies suggest an augmenting antipsychotic effect of estrogen in women.

Part Ten

The Homeless and Schizophrenia

"There was a table set out under the tree ... and the March Hare and the Hatter were having tea at it: a Dormouse was sitting between them, fast asleep, and the other two were using it as a cushion, resting their elbows on it, and talking over its head. 'Very uncomfortable for the Dormouse,' thought Alice, 'only, as it's asleep, I suppose it doesn't mind.'"

Lewis Carroll, *Alice in Wonderland*

88. How prevalent is schizophrenia among the homeless?

Many of us walk and jump over homeless men and woman dressed in multiple layers of old clothes sleeping on city sidewalk-heated grates, not possibly understanding how they could feel and rationalizing that their sleeping souls are oblivious to the cold and pain. The argument given by some is that they prefer living that way and if given housing would choose not to take it. Do we know, however, whether those that are homeless have the capacity to make this decision? Recent research surveys indicate that many of the urban homeless would be diagnosed with schizophrenia. Perhaps *because* of their illness they are incapable of seeking shelter.

Historically, before the rise of public mental institutions run by the states, it was widely known that a large number of homeless individuals lined urban streets, a high percentage of whom had mental illness. It was, in fact, in part for this very reason that psychiatric institutions came into existence in large numbers (detailed in Torrey, 1998). The community mental health center concept that was promoted in the 1960s, combined with the wide-scale use of neuroleptic medication in public psychiatric hospitals, produced a movement for reintegrating these institutionalized people with schizophrenia back into the community. This program, provided for by funds from the federal government in the United States, and similar such projects in other countries established outpatient mental health centers within local communities. These local centers largely failed, however. Primarily, there were not enough community care homes with adequate facilities for patients to be moved to, and the funds provided were inadequate to keep the centers and the corresponding residential facilities maintained. Thus, this so-called worldwide deinstitutionalization came full-circle again to massive increases in homelessness.

Another problem was the lack of coordination of the inpatient care with referral systems to the community mental health centers. Thus, the centers treated many more mildly ill patients who were never before in need of hospitalization, whereas those who were released from the psychiatric hospitals had difficulty becoming integrated into the healthcare system. These newly released patients would then not continue their medication and lose the ability to care for themselves and plan daily living and coping strategies, and so they took to the streets.

Regardless of psychiatric status, people living at or below the federal poverty level are the most vulnerable to experiencing a homeless episode. The estimated annual projections account for 6.3% to 9.6% of the total U.S. population in poverty and 6.2% to 9.3% of children in poverty. Among homeless women in one study, the prevalence of psychiatric disorders was 71%, with substance abuse the leading disorder (43%), followed by anxiety disorders (35%) and then schizophrenia (12%). Many other studies find similar rates for schizophrenia ranging from 2% to 45% internationally and with an average of 11% worldwide, with rates somewhat higher in women than men and higher in the young and the chronically homeless. Suicide rates are also higher in the homeless in general than non-homeless, regardless of psychiatric diagnosis. Another report, *Homelessness: Programs and the People They Serve*, is a recently released set of publications and a collaborative effort of the Census Bureau and the U.S. Department of Housing and Urban Development. Using 1996 statistics, the study's findings are eye opening at the very least. Thirty-eight percent report evidence of alcohol use problems in the past month. Twenty-six percent report drug use problems. Thirty-nine percent report some evidence of mental health problems, and 66% report indicators of one or more of these problems. This report and others are available from the U.S. Department of Housing and Urban Development's Office of Policy Development and Research at 1-800-245-2691 and at this link and address: National Alliance to End Homelessness, (http://www.endhomelessness.org/back/hudreport.ht m), 1518 K Street NW, Suite 206, Washington, DC 20005; 1-202-638-1526; naeh@naeh.org.

89. What causes homelessness?

On a general level, homelessness is caused by poverty and unemployment, but how a person gets to that extreme level and to make the choice to give up and live on a street is more complex. Estimates show that worldwide at least 1.3 million people are homeless, that is, without even basic minimal shelter. Even in a booming economy, at least 2.3 million adults and children, or nearly 1% of the U.S. population, are likely to experience a spell of homelessness at least once during a year. Fleeing from violence was a predominant reason for women to be homeless, which differed markedly from male homelessness. Homelessness in people with schizophrenia has been blamed on a failure of the mental health system to provide adequate care for patients after they are discharged from the hospital. There continues to exist, however, the possibility that the nature of schizophrenia itself and its negative symptoms create homelessness, not for economic reasons, but because these people fail to use cognitive planning abilities to provide themselves with proper shelter, a very basic aspect of human survival.

90. Can homeless people be forced into shelters and hospitals?

Interestingly, a decade ago, many more homeless people were on the streets of New York. What reduced this number so drastically? It was not the better treatment of patients with schizophrenia and/or drug abuse in psychiatric facilities, but it was rather the authority of the mayor of New York, Rudi Giuliani. His goal was to move all of the homeless off the streets and from public parks, building shelters, but mainly using police force to take them off the streets and off of park benches at night, placing them mostly in jails when they did not go to shelters. If a homeless person is not acutely harmful to himself or others, he or she cannot be forced into psychiatric treatment and medication. He or she can, however, be picked up for "loitering" or other crimes and be placed in jail. Often mentally ill persons confined to jail unfortunately do not receive proper medical treatment.

Homelessness remains one of America's most complicated and important social issues. Chronic poverty, coupled with physical and other disabilities, have combined with rapid changes in society, the workplace, and local housing markets to make many people vulnerable to becoming homeless. With the enactment of the Stewart B. McKinney Homeless Assistance Act of 1987, Congress recognized the need to supplement "mainstream" federally funded housing and human services programs with funding that was specifically targeted to assist homeless people. The program instituted includes provisions for emergency shelters, transitional housing programs, permanent housing programs for formerly homeless people, programs distributing vouchers for emergency accommodation, programs accepting vouchers in exchange for giving emergency accommodation, food pantries, soup kitchens, mobile food programs, physical healthcare programs, mental healthcare programs, alcohol/drug programs, HIV/AIDS programs, outreach programs, drop-in centers, and migrant camps that provide emergency shelter for homeless people that seek temporary farming jobs from one state to another (the so-called "migrant workers").

Thus, over the past decade, there has been tremendous growth in services for the homeless. The shelter and housing capacity in the United States within the homeless assistance network grew by 220% between 1988 and 1996, from 275,000 beds to almost 608,000 beds in 1996. Much of the growth is due to new funding and to priorities placed on developing transitional and permanent housing programs for these people. Between 1988 and 1996, the number of such units grew from close to 0 to about 274,000 compared with the capacity of emergency shelters, which grew by only 21%. Soup kitchen and meal distribution services in central cities nearly quadrupled between 1987 and 1996, from 97,000 to 382,100 meals on an average day in winter 1996. Nationally, these programs expected to serve almost 570,000 meals, approximately one third of which were served outside of central cities. Other types of homeless services have also increased, including health services, outreach programs, and drop-in centers.

Part Eleven

Living with Schizophrenia

"Whatever meaning people feel can be derived from their personal suffering, to live without pain would, I believe, be even more meaningful, even more human."

Deepak Chopra (1991), *Unconditional Life: Discovering the Power to Fulfill Your Dreams*

91. What are the origins of the stigma attached to having schizophrenia?

Stigma

literally a "mark"; something visible to others that sets an individual apart from others whether for justified or unjustified reasons.

The word **stigma** dates back to the ancient Greeks who defined this as something unusual about someone's body that suggests something bad and immoral. This term is widely used to be synonymous with something disgraceful or of which to be ashamed. In general, something that is stigmatized is a trait that turns people away from the stigmatized individual, as it is assumed that this person is less than human. Anyone who does not behave within the norms accepted by "society" is stigmatized in a similar manner to minority racial stigmatization. For many decades, families who had affected psychotic individuals would hide them in attics, closets, and basements; this was more easily done in rural than urban settings. There was the fear of a family being stigmatized if one of its members had a mental illness. Until recently, having depression was similar. Over the last decade, however, when individuals who are well respected in the community have gone public with their illnesses (such as Kay Jamison, Mike Wallace, Margot Kidder, Brian Wilson, and others) and published books on the topic, awareness that depression and bipolar disorder are diseases that can be treated has slowly taken place. People with these illnesses may still be stigmatized, but less so than in the past. Public education and awareness have helped to reduce the stigma. It has been less so for schizophrenia, probably because people with this illness do not make good advocates for themselves. Their prominent language and thought disorders, along with residual negative symptoms, prevent them from speaking out and becoming proactive. Thus, it has been up to their families to form public advocacy groups. The many support groups having members coming from well-respected families in the community have helped to establish public networks for regular meeting and education and to lobby for the rights of the disabled mentally ill. With new medications and the return of people with schizophrenia to productive lives and with the knowledge that these are not people to be feared, stigma can be reduced.

92. Can a person with schizophrenia be professionally creative?

Many famous examples of creative people with schizophrenia are available, such as John Nash who received the Nobel Prize for his work on game theory, the artist Van Gogh, or several musicians. Creativity is usually more frequently associated with manic-depressive psychosis than schizophrenia because in mania there is a flurry of grandiose thoughts and an excess of energy, whereas in schizophrenia, there is withdrawal and a loss of internal drive as well as disorganization of thoughts. The latter do not lend themselves to creative products. It is usually the exceptional person (such as John Nash) who was creative prior to having full-blown schizophrenia, but never gets back to that creative state again after the chronic illness sets in, although this is not always the case. John Nash is famous for what he accomplished at a young age before the onset of his psychosis; he was never as productive as he would have been had he not developed schizophrenia.

93. Should I adopt a baby whose birth parent had schizophrenia?

There is a 10-fold or slightly less excess in risk over the general population for a child to develop schizophrenia when a parent has been affected. Thus, adoption of such a child should be treated with caution. The child may appear normal for many years but then tragically become ill after many years of devotion from adoptive parents. The decision is personal but should be considered seriously, at least until medications become available that can be administered early on to prevent a full-blown illness (see Part Four on genetic risk). Adoption agencies should at least now inform prospective families of this history and, if not, the prospective parents should request the information. It may be useful to take this information either to a research psychiatrist who knows genetics for consultation or a genetic counselor who is trained in these issues.

94. Should a person with schizophrenia drive a car?

Reaction tests and simulating driving studies have shown that people with schizophrenia tend not to be able to respond as quickly in a coordinated manner to unexpected changes in driving conditions. Although there are no known statistics on the rates of accidents in people with schizophrenia, you would expect that it could be significantly higher for people with schizophrenia than in the general population. Some statistics show that 50 percent of outpatients with schizophrenia drive automobiles. Antipsychotic medication can affect the ability to drive, although some indication exists that atypical antipsychotics may not have this effect. Nevertheless, providing that a person is not on a sedative medication that causes drowsiness and thus affects driving response, patients with schizophrenia who have been stabilized and are not preoccupied with unsuppressed symptoms are likely responsible drivers on roads that are uncomplicated, short distances, and generally not normally stressful driving stretches. However, under no circumstances should a patient drive when he or she is experiencing an acute episode that is not stabilized with medication. Whether a patient should drive an automobile should be considered on an individual basis. In the future, state driving tests may be modified so that all individuals might be required to take a stimulus-response test. Certainly other medical conditions, such as substance abuse, aging, and other neurological diseases, can hamper driving ability. Schizophrenia should not be singled out.

Part Twelve

Ethical Issues

"*They have said that he was like George Washington and his only crime was his unswerving and uncompromising patriotism, that he was not guilty of treason, that he was not a Fascist, that he was not anti-Semitic, that he was deprived of his rights to a fair trial, and that he was held as a political prisoner. The biggest myth, however, was that he was insane.*"

E. Fuller Torrey (1984) on beginning his book about
Ezra Pound's psychiatric hospitalization

"*The Hadamar gas chamber was set up in the basement.... At the conclusion of the admission procedures the nurse would tell the patients they were to have a nice shower.... The unsuspecting patients would have no objection to such a suggestion ... and the director of the Hadamar center presided over a cocktail party commemorating the killing of their ten-thousandth patient.*"

By Trust Betrayed, Hugh Gregory Gallagher, 1995

95. What does "involuntary" hospital commitment involve?

Many years ago a disgruntled husband could put away his wife for years in a psychiatric hospital. Now, however, there are laws to prevent this. Although the rules of each state and each country vary, in general, when a person is acutely ill and unable to have the capacity to understand what is happening in order to make personal decisions and he or she is considered a danger to himself or others, he or she can be held involuntarily in psychiatric hospitalized treatment for a short period of time, renewable by two physicians. Court hearings can also resolve this if the patients continue to request hospital discharge, but the doctors feel otherwise. Sometimes outpatient commitment is also made mandatory so that patients are required to continue medication even when they do not have insight into the fact that they are ill and in need of the long-term medications. In this case, the only way they would be allowed by law to stay out of the hospital and in the community is if they comply with the court-ordered medication. Sometimes the law can be on the side of the patient who might still be harmful and manage to conceal this behavior. If patients are rational and fail to admit their intentions, there is no way of keeping them in the hospital confined against their will, as was the case with the patient from Long Island who was able to conceal his pathological wish to kill his wife from doctors and nursing staff and left the grounds of Pilgrim State Hospital on a day pass, shortly afterward only to murder his wife.

A related issue is whether a psychiatrist has the responsibility to divulge information received during the doctor–patient relationship if it could imply harm toward another person. One legal issue, known as the Tarasoff Case, arose in California in the mid 1970s. A patient let his doctor know that he felt like harming his wife. Although the doctor called the police who were not trained and did nothing, he failed to warn the intended victim, who was indeed murdered by the patient. This court ruling made it the responsibility of a doctor to warn an intended victim about possible harm. In another case in North Carolina, a psychiatrist was held responsible for a former patient's murderous spree eight months after he was no longer in the psychiatrist's care. A jury found the psychiatrist culpable because when he last saw the patient, the doctor did not follow through to make sure his recommendations for seeking further care and continuing medications were adhered to.

96. What is the legal insanity defense?

An insanity defense is a legal term that excuses people with mental illness from legal responsibility for their crime. Many jurisdictions even allow insanity defenses to be entered on behalf of an offender even when the defendant objects. By far the most frequent psychiatric condition associated with an insanity defense is schizophrenia. Psychiatrists in forming professional opinions about a particular case may need to change their views depending on the actual legal definition, as defined by each jurisdiction. Psychiatrists are not accustomed to this term. Someone can be acutely psychotic but still able to understand the difference between right and wrong actions. Someone may commit a criminal act without understanding his or her actions (e.g., the man who kills his grandparents because "voices" told him to do it and because he "knew" that they were about to kill him or the woman who drove her children into a lake drowning them). Did he or she know that they were doing something wrong? Did the man commit a crime who drove his car through the White House gates because he thought that it was the only way to let the president know his opinions?

Finally, with respect to the release of those people committing a crime who have gone to mental hospitals rather than jail, in New York, an Insanity Defense

Reform Act was passed in 1980 and specified the procedures necessary for releasing persons to the community who were found not guilty of a criminal offense by reason of insanity. The most important condition was participation in an outpatient treatment program. Some follow-up studies, however, have found that one fourth to one third of these patients were rearrested, many for crimes of violence, and others were rehospitalized and their releases revoked. These people obviously constitute a special group of patients that on hospital release need long-term treatment and social guidance in the community with close follow-up.

In some countries, such as in Cuba during the 1970s, and Ireland in the 1800s, as well as other parts of the United Kingdom, the criminally insane were released but were deported to other countries. Although this obviously does not solve the problem for the patients, the country of origin feels healthier.

Interestingly, some surveys actually show that those with psychotic diagnoses, such as schizophrenia, tend to be most of the criminals who obtain insanity defenses, whereas those with a prior criminal history, personality disorders, or drug and alcohol charges tend not to enter insanity pleas. Despite this, there is still a racial disparity so that whites are more likely to be successful with an insanity defense than people from minority backgrounds in the United States. Some thought should be given to such biases.

97. Have there been abuses of the insanity defense?

Many states would like to eliminate the insanity defense because medication may not cure some criminal behavior. After having murdered, a person may not hesitate to do it again. Certainly, John Hinckley, who is on medication and is still in St. Elizabeth's Hospital for having shot President Reagan and stalked a movie star, no longer has the delusions that led him there; nevertheless, aside from home visits, he has never been allowed discharge and will likely live his entire life in the hospital because of the publicity associated with his case and the nature of his delusions to the national political interests.

There have on the other side been historical political abuses of psychiatric diagnoses and the need for hospitalization. During the late 1970s, the World Psychiatric Association was investigating Russian psychiatrists for the hospitalization of political dissidents under the guise of having a particular form of politically invented schizophrenia. More recently, the same practices have been suggested to be taking place in China. Some people have suggested that when Ezra Pound, the poet, was hospitalized at St. Elizabeth's in Washington, DC for many years, it was because of his extreme anti-American political views—not because he was psychotic.

Patient abuses exist as well. Someone who commits a crime can also be astute enough to know that an insanity defense might mean confinement in a psychiatric hospital until the psychiatric condition resolves and then freedom. Thus, symptoms can be mimicked and then resolved. The dilemma is that the only way one can diagnose schizophrenia is by the patient's admission of symptoms and observation of his or her behavior. Sometimes a distinction between malingering and the real illness cannot be ascertained, however, by interviewing a relative or close friend who has observed the patient over time and at other occasions, a more comprehensive picture of the person emerges.

The other side to this issue is that people with mental illness are often placed in prison instead of a psychiatric hospital and then often do not receive the treatment that they need for their illness. Often they have no insight into their illness, and they deny symptoms when prodded. It is only the astute psychiatrist who can tell these two opposite conditions apart. Here is an example of the currently existing problems in prisons when it comes to the management of people with serious mental illness (published in The *New York Times*, February 28, 2005):

> "In City's Jails, Missed Signals Open Way
> to Season of Suicides"
> by Paul von Zielbauer

> *The* New York Times' *year-long examination of Prison Health Services, the biggest commercial provider of medical care to inmates, found instances of disturbing deaths and other troubling treatment.*

> *The warnings were right there in her medical file: a childhood of sexual abuse, a diagnosis of manic depression, a suicide attempt at age 13—all noted when Carina Montes arrived at Rikers Island in September 2002.*

> *State investigators said that none of them were ever seen by the mental health specialist caring for her. He could never track down the file, which by December included another troubling fact: Ms. Montes had been placed on suicide watch by a jail social worker. Not that the suicide watch was terribly reliable; it depended in part on inmates paid 39 cents an hour to check on their suicidal peers.*

> *In her 5 months at Rikers, investigators later discovered that Ms. Montes never saw a psychiatrist.*

> *It did not, however, take a psychiatrist to pick up on the alarms she sounded near the end, when another inmate saw her tearing bedsheets and threatening to kill herself. But the guard who was called had no idea she was on suicide watch, did not notice the sheets and never reported the incident. Six hours later*

Ms. Montes was dead, hanging from a sheet tied to a ventilation grate.

She was 29. Her offense: shoplifting 30 lipsticks.

The death of Carina Montes was one in a spate of suicides in New York City jails in 2003—six in just 6 months, more than in any similar stretch since 1985. None of these people had been convicted of the charges that put them in jail. But in Ms. Montes's death and four of the five others, government investigators reached a stinging judgment about one or both of the authorities responsible for their safety: Prison Health Services, the nation's largest for-profit provider of inmate medical care, and the city correction system. In their reports, investigators faulted a system in which patients' charts were missing, alerts about despondent inmates were lost or unheeded, and neither medical personnel nor correction officers were properly trained in preventing suicide, the leading cause of deaths in American jails.

98. Do patients with schizophrenia have the capacity to give written informed consent for research and other procedures?

Stabilized chronic patients with schizophrenia who are currently functioning outside of a hospital almost always have the capacity to understand the information that is being presented. The question has remained about those who are incapable of living outside of the hospital or who are experiencing an acute psychotic episode. In general, people with schizophrenia still have the capacity to understand instructions if things are explained clearly and slowly, and they are given the opportunity to ask questions. They also have decisional capacity and the ability to exercise their will voluntarily if the time is taken to explain information. Their attention span and preoccupation with their thought disorders and hallucinations during an acute episode makes them appear not to understand. To obtain such evidence of capacity, patients can be explained things carefully and then asked questions to see whether they understood. Also, structured capacity tests can be given to each patient. There is great sensitivity now among legislatures, academicians, researchers, and institutional review boards for human research, and careful rules must be followed to obtain written informed consent from subjects for all kinds of research studies. People who have diseases that reduce their capacity to understand what they are participating in, depending on the nature of a study, can have legal guardians give consent for them. Research progress aimed toward finding better treatments for these disorders is essential; thus, alternative provisions, such as the ability to have a legal guardian to consent who can weigh the risks and benefits carefully, are important. Unfortunately, our country, as well as others, has in its too recent history evidence of abuses by researchers of groups of people who cannot protect their individual rights, such as those who are mentally retarded or demented or those who are prisoners. Thus, legislation has been enacted to safeguard these people from being subject to forceful participation in research.

Another issue is whether someone found mentally ill can be executed for a crime in states that have the death penalty; some state courts have ruled that criminals could not be forcibly medicated in order to make them competent for involuntary execution.

99. Can genetic information be abused?

In Part Six on genetics, some of the eugenic movement was described. Psychiatrists were prominent in using superficial genetic statistics to suggest that sterilizing and then exterminating people who had "inherited" mental illness would be best for society. We need to proceed cautiously given the historical potential for use of genetic information to scapegoat religious and other groups. Many other possibilities of abuse of genetic information are looming in the future, since with advanced technology, we can now determine the variants of genes that are present in embryos. What harm will we be doing in the future if certain variants are not allowed to continue according to the rules of evolution and natural selection? The movie *Gattaca* was provocative and went relatively unnoticed. It was a startling look at what could happen in the future. The main characters in *Gattaca* were a "genetically enhanced" population of people who discriminated against those who were born by natural unions of men and women. This may be more of a reality, given today's technology, than simply science fiction. Other abuses have to do with the public use of genetic information if it is known at birth. Could insurance companies and life insurance salespersons refuse to insure individuals for medical care or life who have inherited the probability of getting certain diseases? Will there be job discrimination, education discrimination, etc.? Instead of the current cultural, ethnic, and racial discrimination, a new form of "genetic" discrimination could occur. These are all things to be prepared for and to govern against by legislation.

100. What support groups, books, and websites can I go to for help?

A list of support groups, websites, and books can be found under Resources.

This book has been about public awareness of schizophrenia and is written so that the abuses based only on scientific half-truths will not occur. Schizophrenia is on the extreme edge of the wide range of what the world calls "normality," whatever it is defined in each culture and at each point in time. It is an illness, however, by virtue of the pain and destruction it causes to those afflicted. With the eventual development of future medications that target its biology, this illness has the hope of being prevented. No one should feel shame or be stigmatized because he or she suffers from schizophrenia, rather he or she should receive the best treatment from those who are trained to give it and then live their lives to their best potential.

Resources

Support Groups

The most prominent support group in the United States is the National Alliance for the Mentally Ill (NAMI), which has local chapters throughout the United States. The national office is located at Colonial Place Three, 2107 Wilson Boulevard, Suite 300, Arlington, VA 22201-3042; 1-703-524-7600 or www.NAMI.org.

In the United Kingdom, the largest support group is Schizophrenia, a National Emergency (SANE), which is at 1st Floor Cityside House, 40 Adler Street, London, E1 1EE; 020-7375-1002, london@sane.org.uk, and www.sane.org.uk.

The following books that provide further information about schizophrenia and related disorders can provide comfort for families, friends, and individuals who have been diagnosed with schizophrenia. A more complete reference list appears on the next page.

Similar organizations exist in other countries as well.

Recommended Books

Andreasen NC (2001). *Brave New Brain: Conquering Mental Illness in the Era of the Genome*. Oxford: Oxford University Press.

Jamison KR (1995). *An Unquiet Mind: A Memoir of Mood and Madness*. New York: Alfred A. Knopf.

Jamison KR (1999). *Night Falls Fast: Understanding Suicide*. New York: Alfred A. Knopf.

Torrey EF (2001). *Surviving Schizophrenia: A Manual for Families, Consumers, and Providers*, 4th ed. New York: Quill.

Torrey EF (1998). *Out of the Shadows: Confronting America's Mental Illness Crisis*, 2nd ed. New York: John Wiley & Sons.

Recomended Investigations

Home movies taken by Elaine Walker, Atlanta while investigating delayed motor development in people who later develop schizophrenia.

Recommended Websites

National Institute of Mental Health website:
http://www.nimh.nih.gov/healthinformation/schizophreniamenu.cfm
or
http://www.nimh.nih.gov/publicat/schizsoms.cfm
If, for some reason, these links do not work, try the NIMH home page at http://www.nimh.nih.gov/.
National Alliance for Research on Schizophrenia and Depression (NARSAD): www.NARSAD.org

References

American Psychiatric Association (2000). *Diagnostic and Statistical Manual of Mental Disorders*, 4th ed., text revision (DSM-IV-TR). Washington, DC: American Psychiatric Association Press.

Andreasen NC (2001). *Brave New Brain: Conquering Mental Illness in the Era of the Genome*. Oxford: Oxford University Press.

Aschaffenburg G (ed.). (1911-1928). Dementia praecox oder die Gruppe der Schizofrenien. *Handbuch der Psychiatrie*. Leipzig and Vienna.

Bak M, Myin-Germeys I, Hanssen M, Bijl R, Vollebergh W, Delespaul P, van Os J (2003). When does experience of psychosis result in a need for care? A prospective general population study. *Schizophr Bull* 29(2):349–358.

Chopra D (1991). *Unconditional Life: Discovering the Power to Fulfill Your Dreams*. New York: Bantam Books.

Crow TJ (1990). The continuum of psychosis and its genetic origins. *Br J Psychiatry* 156:788–797.

Crow TJ (1997). Is schizophrenia the price that Homo sapiens pays for language? *Schizophr Res* 28:127–141.

Crow TJ (2000). Schizophrenia as the price that Homo sapiens pays for language: A resolution of the central paradox in the origin of the species. *Brain Res Brain Res Rev* 31:118–129.

DeLisi LE (ed.). (1990). *Depression in Schizophrenia*. Washington, DC: American Psychiatric Association Press.

DeLisi LE (2000). Unifying the concept of psychosis through brain morphology. In: Maneros A, Angst J (eds.). (2000). *Bipolar Disorders: 100 Years After Manic Depressive Insanity*. The Netherlands: Kluwer.

DeLisi LE (2001). Speech disorder in schizophrenia: Review of the literature and new study of the relation to uniquely human capacity for language. *Schizophr Bull* 27:481–496.

DeLisi LE, Crow TJ. (1989). Evidence for an X chromosome locus for schizophrenia. *Schizophr Bull* 15:431–440.

El-Hai J (2004) *The Lobotomist: A Maverick Medical Genius and His Tragic Quest to Rid the World of Mental Illness.* Hoboken, NJ: John Wiley & Sons.

Faulks S (2005) *Human Traces.* Hutchinson, The Random House Group, Ltd., London, UK.

Fink M (1999). *Electroshock: Healing Mental Illness.* Oxford: Oxford University Press.

Geller JL, Harris M (1994). *Women of the Asylum.* New York: Doubleday Anchor Books.

Gottesman II (1991). *Schizophrenia Genesis: The Origins of Madness.* New York: WH Freeman.

Gottesman II, Shields J (1982). *Schizophrenia: The Epigenetic Puzzle.* Cambridge: Cambridge University Press.

Gould SJ (1981). *The Mismeasure of Man.* New York: W.W. Norton and Company.

Henig RM (2000). *The Monk in the Garden.* Boston: Houghton Mifflin.

Isaac RJ, Armat VC (2000). *Madness in the Streets : How Psychiatry and the Law Abandoned the Mentally Ill.* Treatment Advocacy Center.

Jamison KR (1995). *An Unquiet Mind: A Memoir of Mood and Madness.* New York: Alfred A. Knopf.

Jamison KR (1999). *Night Falls Fast: Understanding Suicide.* New York: Alfred A. Knopf.

Johnstone EC, Crow TJ, Frith DC, Husband J, Krel L (1976). Cerebral ventricular size and cognitive impairment in schizophrenia. *Lancet* 2:924–926.

Kasanetz EF (1979). Tecnica per investigare il ruolo di fattori ambientale sulla genesi della schizophrenia. *Riv Psicol Anal* 10:193–202.

Kety SS, Rosenthal D, Wender PH, Schulsinger F (1968). The types and prevalences of mental illness in the biological and adoptive families of adopted schizophrenics. In Rosenthal D, Kety SS (eds.). *The Transmission of Schizophrenia*. Oxford: Pergammon, 345–362.

Kingdon DG, Turkington D (June 1, 1995). *Cognitive Behavioral Therapy for Schizophrenia*, new ed. Psychology Press.

Kraepelin E (1907). *Etiology of Dementia Praecox, Lehrbuch Der Psychitarie*, 7th ed. 1907.

Menninger KA (1926). Influenza and schizophrenia: An analysis of post-influenzal "dementia praecox" as of 1918 and five years later. *Am J Psychiatry* 5:469–529.

Nasar S (1998). *A Beautiful Mind*. New York: Simon and Schuster.

Nasrallah HA, Smeltzer DJ (2003). *Contemporary Diagnosis and Management of the Patient with Schizophrenia*. Handbooks in Healthcare Company.

Reeder, C and Wykes T (2005). Cognitive Remediation Therapy for Schizophrenia. Routledge, London.

Rosenthal D (ed.). (1963). *The Genain Quadruplets: A Case Study and Theoretical Analysis of Heredity and Environment in Schizophrenia*. New York: Basic Books.

Rosenthal D, Wender PH, Kety SS, Welner J, Schulsinger F (1968). Schizophrenic's offspring reared in adoptive homes. In: Rosenthal D, Kety SS (eds.). *The Transmission of Schizophrenia*. Oxford: Pergammon, 377–391.

Torrey EF (1980). *Schizophrenia and Civilization*. New York: Aronson.

Torrey EF (1984). *The Roots of Treason: Ezra Pound and the Secret of St. Elizabeth's*. New York: McGraw-Hill Book Company.

Torrey EF (1988). *Nowhere to Go: The Tragic Odyssey of the Homeless Mentally Ill*. New York: Harper & Row.

Torrey EF (1998). *Out of the Shadows: Confronting America's Mental Illness Crisis*, 2nd ed. New York: John Wiley & Sons.

Torrey EF (2001). *Surviving Schizophrenia: A Manual for Families, Consumers, and Providers*, 4th ed. New York: Quill.

Torrey EF, Miller J (2001). *The Invisible Plague: The Rise of Mental Illness from 1750 to the Present*. New Brunswick, NJ: Rutgers University Press.

Torrey EF, Peterson MR (1976). The viral hypothesis of schizophrenia. *Schizophr Bull* 2:136–146.

Verdoux H, van Os J (2002). Psychotic symptoms in non-clinical populations and the continuum of psychosis. *Schizophr Res* 54:59–65.

Glossary

Alzheimer's disease: This is one of a few progressive brain diseases that has been more frequently diagnosed recently in older people who appear disoriented and have difficulty communicating properly with others. It consists of specific characteristic changes in the brain that can be seen only by autopsy after death, but MRI scans can also be revealing. The usual signs that will appear are large ventricles and atrophy of a region of the brain crucial for remembering, the hippocampus. Other parts of the brain can also be affected. Thus, a person with Alzheimer's disease has trouble remembering what happened one minute ago and has difficulty forming sentences and speaking, eventually progressing into not being able to take care of his or her basic needs.

Antipsychotic: Any medication that specifically suppresses the positive symptoms of hallucinations and delusions. This medication can also be useful in other conditions as a strong tranquilizer.

Bipolar affective disorder: A psychiatric condition characterized by mood swings that occur episodically. Sometimes, particularly when very "high" (manic), people with bipolar disorder can have many of the characteristic positive symptoms of schizophrenia.

Catatonia: A condition that is characterized by extremes in behavior, of which the individual appears to be unaware. These behaviors include being mute or in a stupor and immobile to, at the other extreme, being in an excitatory state of an extreme frenzy or agitated excitement. This condition is not specific to schizophrenia; however, when it is periodically present in someone who has other characteristics of schizophrenia, it is then diagnosed as the subtype called "catatonic schizophrenia."

Catatonic Behavior: Behavior characterized by muscular tightness or rigidity and lack of response to the environment.

Chromosome: A structure present in the nucleus of every cell of the body of any living thing containing genes. It is shaped like a long cylinder separated into two arms that are held together in the approximate middle by a structure called the centromere. The two arms have been named "p" and "q" arms, and the length of the cylinder has been quantified by the distance from the distal tip of the "p" arm. The "p" arm is usually the shorter of the two chromosome arms. The total distance of one chromosome is measured in "centimorgans," named after the scientist who worked out the method for measuring it, Morgan. In addition, people who view chromosomes under the microscope have noticed differences in the dark and light constitutions of the chromosome that may mean breaks in where clusters of genes start and end. Thus, a method was developed for counting these bands. The band numbers begin from the centromere and go distally, using consecutively higher numbers on each arm. These two methods of measuring chromosomes and their size then gives geneticists the ability to know where different genes are located on the chromosome. Thus, when a gene is located on chromosome 6q21, 150 cM from pter this means it is on the sixth chromosome on the larger arm (the "q" arm) and within the 21st band down that arm. Its exact distance from the distal tip of the "p" arm is 150 centimorgans. More and more information given to the public will now talk in these terms, for example: "A gene for XX disease has been found by researchers on chromosome 6q21."

Cognition: The quality of the mind that allows animals to think, reason, and manipulate their environment to survive. Cognition can be measured by psychological tests. Of course, the tests are much simpler for nonhuman animals and are most complicated for humans. The well-known IQ is one measure of human cognition.

Cognitive behavioral therapy (CBT): This is a brief form of psychotherapy based on the principle that the way one thinks about something causes actions. Thus, it is focused on changing thinking patterns that lead to disruptive behavior. Several different techniques are available for this. This form of therapy is used for a variety of psychiatric disorders. Unlike the way it sounds, this is not a type of therapy that trains people to improve their cognition or intellectual abilities.

Command hallucinations: Imaginary voices that tell the hearer what to do.

Computed tomography (CT): A form of X-ray that is able to view the brain in more detail than a standard skull X-ray. However, it has been largely replaced by MRI as a diagnostic technique to examine details of the brain. The advantage CT has over MRI is that it detects bone change, whereas MRI views the brain tissue, and is not sensitive to bone.

Cortex (cerebral cortex): The outer portion of the brain. It consists mostly of the "gray matter" that contains nerve cells.

Delusion: A false belief based on faulty judgment about one's environment.

Depression: A major psychiatric condition characterized by profound sadness all day. It is usually accompanied by physical symptoms, such as loss of appetite, loss of sleep, and slowness in movements and speech. If the condition continues as long as one week without relief and interferes with a person's ability to function, it is then called major depression.

Disorganizational syndrome: A set of symptoms related to general disorganization (speech and/or behavioral disorganization).

DNA: DNA is made of different nucleic acids: adenine, guanine, thiamine, and cytosine and is put together in the form of a triple helical structure. The variation in genes between individuals depends on the sequence of these nucleic acids in an individual's genes. DNA makes up the reproducing portion (i.e., genes) of chromosomes in animals and plants and makes up many viruses.

Dopamine: A chemical substance that is important for conveying "messages" between nerve cells in the brain.

DSM-IV: The diagnostic and statistical manual developed by leading clinical psychiatrists in the United States for the systematic evaluation of psychiatric patients and assigning diagnoses to groups of symptoms. There have been four major separate revisions of this code of diagnoses since its inception. It has two axes: Axis I is for major diagnoses, and Axis II is for personality disorders.

Dyskinesia: Difficulty in performing movements voluntarily.

Electroconvulsive therapy: A type of treatment usually for depression that gives a series of electrical shocks to regions of the brain given in sessions that are separated by several days. The way it exerts its effects is unknown. However, it is not dangerous or painful and is accompanied by an anesthetic when administered. The only known side effect is memory loss subsequent to the treatment.

Electroencephalogram (EEG): A type of test whereby electrodes are placed on several areas of the head and recordings are made of the brain's electrical activity.

Enzymes: Proteins in the body that digest other substances through biochemical reactions. They are the "tools" of metabolism.

Estrogen: A female hormone that is produced in the female organs (ovaries). It is produced in different amounts throughout the menstrual cycle and is reduced after menopause.

Family therapy: Any of several therapeutic approaches in which a family is treated as a whole.

Fecundity: Bearing children.

Fertility: Having the normal biology that gives one the ability to bear children.

Fish oil: 3-Omega fatty acids. These are substances important for the building of the lining of nerves. For good functioning of the nervous system, it is important that these fatty acids are in abundance. This is a commercial product that can be bought in health food stores at various levels of purity and has been advertised as a "cure-all" for many conditions; most claims have not been substantiated scientifically.

Functional MRI: A brain scan that shows actions taking place in the brain in response to a stimulus. The stimulus could be anything, such as voluntary movement of the fingers to memorizing a set of words.

Gene: A functional unit of heredity that is in a fixed place in the structure of a chromosome.

Geneticists: Scientists who study the inheritance of traits in humans, animals, or plants.

Glutaimine / Glutamate: An amino acid that is a building block of proteins. It is also by itself a major neurotransmitter in the brain (i.e., transmits information from cell to cell); by stimulating the activity of the cells, it excites them into activity.

Gray matter: The brownish-gray nerve tissue of the brain and spinal cord that contains the nerve cells.

Hallucinations: Experiencing something from any of the five senses that is not occurring in reality (e.g., hearing voices when no one is there to speak, seeing images of things that are not really there, smelling something that is not there, feeling something touch one's body when it is not actually there, or tasting something that one is not eating).

Hippocampus: This relatively small brain structure lies deep within the temporal lobe and is thought to be crucial for memory. It has been given this name because of its unusual shape.

Homo sapiens: The scientific designation for modern human beings.

Immunoglobulins: The proteins that help the body respond to foreign substances and infections.

Insanity: Mental malfunctioning or unsoundness of mind to produce lack of judgment and to the degree that the individual cannot determine right from wrong.

Intermediate phenotype: This is sometimes also called an "endophenotype." It is the trait in genetic terms that a gene is responsible for producing whatever makes a person more vulnerable to getting an illness. For example, an intermediate phenotype for schizophrenia may be a change in the structure of the brain that in turn may put someone at risk to get schizophrenia.

Linkage: A genetic term that signifies a relationship between two or more genes on the same chromosome that are relatively close together so that sometimes the variations in the traits that each represents are inherited together in the same individual.

Lobotomy: The surgical division of one or more brain tracts. It is usually referred to as cutting nerves that run from the frontal lobe to the thalamus in the brain. It has been done in various ways, most often by inserting a needle above the nose in between the eyes. This serves to disconnect nerves connecting the frontal lobe of the brain to other structures.

Magnetic resonance imaging: A method to examine the tissue of the brain using a magnetic field and computer system. The machine itself consists of a horizontal tube inside of a giant magnet. The patient having an MRI scan lies on his or her back and slides into the tube on a special table. After inside, the patient is scanned.

Magnetic resonance spectroscopy: A type of MRI scan that examines chemical spectras in the brain. These chemicals are those that are present in the structure of membranes or metabolic activity in nerve cells and between cells.

Manic behavior: Feeling excessively elated and cheery with very fast speech and thoughts.

Microarray: This is an orderly arrangement of DNA samples to identify many genes at one time. They can contain thousands of genes on one small plate or "chip." An experiment with a single DNA chip or microarray can provide researchers information on thousands of genes simultaneously.

Monozygotic twins: Twins born at the same time who originate from the splitting of the same egg after it has been fertilized. The DNA is identical in both twins; and thus the twins are sometimes referred to as identical.

Negative symptoms: Those characteristics of psychiatric illness that present as withdrawn behavior, an expressionless face, a lack of initiative, a lack of interest, slow speech, and not saying much when talking, slowed thoughts, and slowed movements. Sometimes these symptoms are confused with either depression or side effects of medication.

Neurodevelopmental: Happening during the growth and formation of different structures of the brain.

Neuroleptic: Any medication that when given to animals will cause catalepsy. This name then was used to label all drugs that had an effect on reducing the symptoms of schizophrenia. They are sometimes known as the "major tranquilizers."

Neuroleptic Malignant Syndrome: This is a severe, although rare, side effect of neuroleptic treatment and its cause is unknown. It begins with rigidity or worsening in psychiatric symptoms despite increases in medication. Some of the warning signs are fast heart beat, high fluctuating blood pressure, tremors, sweating, and fever. Cessation of neuroleptic therapy is the only treatment. This is a serious medical emergency that requires immediate treatment.

Paranoid: Excessive or irrational suspicion or distrust of others.

Pharmacotherapy: Treatment of disease through the use of drugs.

Phenotype: The trait that is expressed by a gene. For example, having blue eyes or brown eyes would be phenotypes.

Pneumoencephalography: An X-ray picture of the brain taken by injection of air into the cerebral ventricular space. This was a method used to detect whether a patient had brain atrophy prior to the invention of computed tomography and magnetic resonance imaging. This method is no longer in use.

Positive symptoms: Considered the active symptoms of hallucinations and delusions of schizophrenia.

Positron emission tomography (PET Scanning): This is a radiologic procedure that measures the metabolism of a radiolabeled substance that is injected into a subject's vein and one that is known to enter the brain relatively rapidly. Pictures are then taken of the brain with the regions metabolizing the injected substance "lighting-up." PET scans are valuable tools to detect early brain tumors and have been useful in Alzheimer's

research. However, they are difficult and expensive to perform, requiring a cyclotron to manufacture the radiolabeled compound and are also uncomfortable for patients. Thus, they have not been popular in recent years among schizophrenia researchers.

Premorbid: The time period before any symptoms of a disorder, including subtle signs, have developed.

Prenatal: The period between conception and birth.

Prodrome: An early or premonitory symptom of a disease. If true specific prodromal symptoms are known, one can detect the illness early. These symptoms signify that the disease will be almost certain.

Psychotherapy: The treatment of mental or emotional problems by psychological means.

Psychotic: People are considered psychotic if they have lost touch with reality, have delusions (i.e., false beliefs), and hallucinations. They often are exhibiting bizarre and risky behavior and do not seem to be aware that they are doing anything unusual.

Residual: Having some nonspecific symptoms (usually negative symptoms), but no longer active psychotic ones.

Schizoaffective: Having both prominent symptoms of schizophrenia and depression and/or mania that overlap with the schizophrenia-like symptoms. However, they do not always coincide, so that sometimes the patients have only schizophrenia-like symptoms and at other times, although less so, only mania or depressive symptoms.

Schizophrenia: Any of a group of psychotic disorders usually characterized by withdrawal from reality, illogical patterns of thinking, delusions, and hallucinations, and accompanied in varying degrees by other emotional, behavioral, or intellectual disturbances. Schizophrenia is associated with dopamine imbalances in the brain and defects of the frontal lobe and is caused by genetic, other biological, and psychosocial factors.

Schizophreniform: Having the symptoms of schizophrenia, but too early in the course of illness to tell whether the symptoms are of a schizophrenia illness.

Serotonin: A hormone found in the brain, platelets, digestive tract, and pineal gland. It acts both as a neurotransmitter (a substance that nerves use to send messages to one another) and a vasoconstrictor (a substance that causes blood vessels to narrow). A lack of serotonin in the brain is thought to be a cause of depression.

Sickle-cell anemia: An inherited disease in which the red blood cells, normally disc-shaped, become crescent shaped.

Stigma: Literally a "mark"; something visible to others that sets an individual apart from others whether for justified or unjustified reasons.

Superior temporal gyrus: A portion of the temporal lobe of the brain that has many functions related to language, including hearing it and speaking it.

Tranquilizer: Any drug that is used to calm or pacify an anxious and/or agitated person. There are minor and major classes of tranquilizers that have different chemical properties and are indicated for different psychiatric conditions, the minor ones for anxiety in a person who has not lost a sense of reality but who needs calming. Major tranquilizers are the class of drugs used for psychotic symptoms.

Ventricles: As this term applies to the brain, the spaces connecting throughout the brain that provide a system for the circulation of the fluid present in the brain called cerebrospinal fluid. The ventricles in the brain consist of the lateral ventricles, third and fourth ventricles and connect to the spinal column and bathe the spinal cord.

White matter: Whitish brain and spinal cord tissue composed mostly of nerve fibers and its shiny protective coat called myelin.

Working memory: This is a more contemporary term for short-term memory. It is thought of as an active system for temporarily storing and manipulating information needed for conducting complex tasks such as learning, reasoning, and comprehending things. There are two components of working memory: storage and central executive functions. The two storage systems within working memory are for temporary storage of verbal and visual information. The central executive function is thought to be a process that is very active and responsible for the selection, initiation, and termination of processing the storing and retrieving of memories.

Index

A

Abilify (aripiprazole), 34
Adoption, 111–112. *See also* Genetic risk
    factors; Studies
Alcohol, use of, 4, 84, 89–90, 105
Alzheimer's Disease, 20
Artane, 36
Atypicals. *See* Drugs

B

Bipolar affective disorder, 11–12, 20, 110
Birth complications, 46
Brain, 46, 95, 96, 101. *See also* Hoffer, Dr.
    Abram; Studies
    abnormalities / differences / changes in,
        12, 66–67, 72
    and ECT, 42
    and EEG, 56
    and schizophrenia, 6, 18–19, 20
    conditions that mimic schizophrenia, 22
    lobotomy(ies), 32–33
    nicotine in, 85
    postmortem, 51, 54, 64
Breast-feeding, 101

C

Catatonia, 6, 12–13
CATIE, 35

CBT (Cognitive behavioral therapy), 27,
    36–38
Chemical imbalance, 76–77
Cigarette smoking, excessive, 84–85
Clozapine, 18, 33–34, 95
Cogentin, 20, 36
Cognition, 15, 20
Community mental health centers, 15,
    104–105
Consent, written informed, 119–120
Creativity, 111
Crimes, 89, 91, 107, 116

D

Delusion(s), 4–6, 67, 101, 116–117. *See also*
    Hallucinations
    as distinguished from "excessive
        religiosity," 17
    as positive symptoms, 18, 33
    in bipolar disorder, 11–12
    in schizoaffective disorder, 10–11
    voices, 16–17
Depression, 9, 19–20, 95, 110
    manic, 10, 12, 118
    negative symptoms, 6, 18
    postpartum, 100–101
    Serotonin / SSRIs, 77, 96
    suicide, leading to, 94, 118
    therapy for, 37, 42–43

Diet / dietary supplements, 22, 36, 38–39
Disorganizational syndrome, 5
DNA testing, 68
Dopamine hypothesis, 77
Driving, 112
Drug / treatment trials, 34–35, 38–40,
    98–99, 102
Drugs. *See also* Medication(s)
    atypicals, 18, 34–36
    neuroleptic(s), 10, 34, 77–78, 98–101,
        104
    new(er), 13, 34, 43, 69
    pharmacogenetics, 68
    pharmacotherapy, 27
    street, 4, 10, 82–83, 94
DSM-IV, 4
Dyskinesia, tardive, 21, 34, 35

E

ECT (Electroconvulsive therapy), 42–43
EEG (Electroencephalogram), 56, 76
Estrogen, role in suppressing symptoms, 99,
    102
Ethical concerns, in the handling of genetic
    data, 69
Eugenics, 54
Evening primrose oil/GLA (gamma-
    linolenic acid), 39

F

Family, 30, 33, 99, 102, 110
    and violence, 88–89
    bad relationships, 48–49, 98
    physician, 9, 26
    studies, 43, 44, 56–57, 59–60, 91
        genetic, 61, 63, 69
    support, 14, 94, 95, 101
    therapy, 27, 40–41
Federal government, 15, 29, 104, 118–119
Fertility/fecundity, 22–23
Fish oils, 38

G

Genain Quadruplets, 55–57
Genetic origin, 23–24. *See also* Genetic risk
    factors
Genetic risk factors, 53–69, 79, 111
Genetic testing, ethical concerns, 69,
    120–121

Geodon (ziprasidone), 34
GLA (gamma-linolenic acid), 39
Glutamate, 65, 66, 77–78

H

Haldol, 34, 35
Hallucinations, 4–5, 67, 119–120. *See also*
    Delusions
    auditory, 9, 16–17, 22, 43
    command, 16, 90, 95
    positive symptoms, 18, 33
Hippocampus, 46, 74–75
History, xiii, xiv
    adoption, 112
    birth complications, 46–47, 100
    care for the mentally ill, 15, 31–32
    forced participation in research, 120
    genetics vs. "Eugenics," 54–55
    involuntary hospitalization of women,
        98
    isolation from society, 31
    of violence, 88, 90
Hoffer, Dr. Abram, 39
Homelessness, 104–108
Horobin, David, 39

I

Informed consent, written, 119–120
Insanity defense, 115–117
Insurance coverage, 27–29, 37, 69, 121
Involuntary commitment / execution, 98,
    114–115, 120
IQ, 15, 20–21

J

Jail(s), 9, 91–92, 107, 115. *See also* Prisons
    suicide in, 118–119
    the homeless, 106–107

L

Language problems, 18–19, 24, 42, 47–48,
    67, 110
Legal insanity defense, 115–117
Living environments, 15, 29, 49–50. *See also*
    Homelessness
Lobotomy (ies), 30, 32–33

M

Manic behavior / manic depression, 10–12, 42, 111, 118
Marijuana, as causal, 82–83
Medication(s), 14, 21, 27–28, 30, 41. *See also* Drugs; Treatment
  alternative, 38–40
  and alcohol consumption, 84
  and CBT, 36
  and cigarette smoking, 85
  and criminal behavior, 116
  and driving, 112
  and marijuana use, 83
  and pregnancy, 99
  and suicide attempts, 94–95
  and the homeless, 104–105, 107
  and violence, 88–92
  antipsychotic / Clozapine, 33–34, 95
  estrogen, 102
  glycine and d-serine, 78
  in adopted children, 111
  mandatory, 114–115
  neuroleptic, 10, 15, 76–77
    and Cogentin, 20
    and street drugs, 9–10
    history of, 31
  new / future, 68, 110, 122
  positive and negative symptoms, 6, 18, 78
  response in women, 98, 99–102
  side effects, 16, 35–36
  with ECT, 42–43
Mellaril, 34
Memory problems, 20
Methamphetamine(s), 83
Microarray, 63–64
Motherhood, 46–48, 100–102
MRI / MRS scans, 20, 75–76, 79
Muscular problems. *See* Dyskinesia, tardive

N

NAMI (National alliance for the mentally ill), 29, 44
Navane, 34
Negative symptoms, 4, 6, 18–20, 78, 106, 110
Neurodevelopmental hypothesis, 79
Neuroleptics. *See* Drugs
Nongenetic risk factors, 45–51

O

Occupational therapy, 28, 95
Orthomolecular therapy, 27

P

Paranoid, 5–6, 8, 26, 94
  schizophrenia, 88, 90, 98
Parity, in health care, 29
PCP, 77–78, 82–83
PET (positron emission tomography) scans, 77
Pharmacogenetics, 68
Pharmacotherapy, 27, 41, 98
Phenotype (endophenotype), intermediate, 66–67
Pneumoencephalography, 73
Positive symptoms, 5, 11, 18, 19, 33, 78
Postpartum relapse, 100–101
Pregnancy, 46, 51, 99–100
Premorbid, 12, 14, 21, 94
Prison(s). *See also* Jails
  Prison Health Services, 117–119
  safeguards against forceful participation in research, 120
Prodrome / Prodromal stage, 4, 27, 36
Psychopathology, 17, 84
Psychotherapy, 6, 27, 37, 40
Psychotic behavior, 4, 30, 47, 110
  and Clozapine, 34
  and depressive behavior, 95
  episodes, 38, 49, 55, 98, 119
  states, 16–17
  symptoms, 11, 13, 20

R

Religiosity, excessive, 5, 16–17
Religious sects, 47, 121
Research. *See also* Research studies
  "expressed emotion," 48
  biologic, 12, 72–79
  CBT (cognitive behavioral therapy), 36–37
  diet, 38
  excessive cigarette smoking, 84–85
  genetic, 60–62, 65, 69, 112
  GLA (gamma-linolenic acid), 39
  IQ, 20
  lack of, 23, 38, 41, 48
  microarray technology, 63–64

MRI/MRS, 75–76, 79
psychiatric, 8
the homeless, 104–106
twins, 58
violent behavior, predicting, 89
Research studies, 19, 38, 43, 44, 119–120.
    See also Genain Quadruplets;
    Research; Studies
and women, 99, 100–102
Residual stage, 4
and negative symptoms, 18, 41, 110
subtype, 6
symptoms, 10, 17, 41, 110

S

Schizoaffective disorder, 10, 11, 20, 98
Schizophrenia. *See also* Split personality
abuse of genetic information, 120–121
alcohol and cigarettes, use of, 84–85
and adoption, 111
and homelessness, 104–108
and neuroleptics, 10
as "chemical imbalance," 76–77
catatonic, 13
causes, 46–47, 50–51 (*See also* Genetic
    risk factors)
    bad family relationships, 48–49
    birth complications, 46–47
    diet, 38–40
    drug use, 82–83
    genetic / chances of inheriting,
        23–24, 54–69, 82, 99
    in cultural and racial groups, 47–48
    in immigrants, 49
    marijuana use, 83
    neurodevelopmental hypothesis, 79
    rural *vs.* urban living, 49–50
    viruses / infection, 50–51
celebrities, who suffer from
    Brian Wilson, xv, 110
    Joan of Arc, xv
    John Hinckley, Jr., xiv, 88, 116
    John Nash, xv, 3, 111
    Kay Jamison, 25, 110
    King Christian 7 of Denmark, xv, 7
    Margot Kidder, 38, 110
    Mike Wallace, 110
    the Unabomber (Ted Kaczynski),
        xv, 88
    the Yorkshire Ripper, xv, 88

Van Gogh, xv, 111
conditions that mimic, 11, 22, 75
course, of illness, 14–15, 22
    depression, experiencing, 19, 95
    early, 10, 33
    preventing, 43
    progressive, 72
creativity, effect on, 111
defined, 4–6, 11, 12, 15, 23–24, 48
development of, 8–9, 21, 83, 95, 99
diagnosis of, 17, 47, 89, 91, 94
driving, 112
drugs that mimic symptoms of, 77–78,
    83
history of treatment, 31–32
in children, 19, 57–60
in women, 98–102
informed consent, written, 119–120
insurance coverage, 27–29, 37, 69, 121
involuntary commitment / execution,
    30, 98, 114–115, 120
legal insanity defense, 115–117
living with, 110–112
neurodevelopmental hypothesis, 79
possible effects of
    reduced lifespan, 21–22
    reduced offspring, 22–23
signs, 7, 9, 18, 26–27
suicidal thoughts, 94–95
support groups, 121–123
symptoms
    depression, 19–20
    differences in the brain, 72–74
    excessive religiosity, 17
    language problems, 18–19, 24, 42,
        47–48, 67, 110
    low IQ, 21
    memory problems, 20
    muscular problems, 21
    positive and negative, 18–19, 78
    violence, 88–91
    voices, 4, 16, 90, 95, 115
tests for, 72–76
treatment by professionals, 26–28
Schizophreniform, 10
Seroquel (quetiapine), 34
Serotonin, 77, 95–96
Social workers, 26, 27, 28, 40
Split personality, 6
SSRIs (Serotonin receptor uptake
    inhibitors), 95–96

Stigma, 15, 35, 69, 110–111, 122
Street drugs. *See* Drugs
Studies. *See also* Genain Quadruplets
  adoption, 56, 58
  bad family relationships, 48–49
  birth complications, 46
  brain, 73–79
  CBT (cognitive behavioral therapy),
    36–37
  children who later develop
    schizophrenia, 19, 21
  chromosomal linkage, 61–64
  criminal behavior, 91
  criminally insane, recidivism rate after
    release, 115–116
  cultural or racial groups, 47
  diet, 36, 38–40
  driving, 112
  drug side effects, 35
  ECT (electroconvulsive therapy), 42–43
  estrogen, antipsychotic effect in women,
    99, 102
  evening primrose oil, 39–40
  family, 57, 59, 91
  fertility/fecundity, 22–23
  genetic, 60, 61, 63–69
  homelessness, 105
  immigrants, 49
  informed consent, written, 119–120
  marijuana use, 83
  memory / IQ, 20–21
  microarray, 63–67
  of women, 99–102
  participation in, 43–44
  twins, 56–61
  viruses, as cause of schizophrenia, 50–51
  World Health Association /
    Organization, 23, 47
Suicide, 7, 8
  prevention of, 119
  prison system, as causal, 118–119
  rates, 22, 105
  suicidal behavior, 94–95
  threatening, 91
  when most likely to occur, 10

T
Tests, 72, 120
  driving, 112
  EEG, 76

  psychological, 15, 20
Therapy(ies)
  CBT (cognitive behavioral therapy), 27,
    36–37
  ECT (electroconvulsive therapy), 42–43
  family, 27, 40–41
  older, 31–32, 84
  orthomolecular, 27
  pharmacotherapy, 27, 41
    in women, 98
  psychotherapy, 6, 27, 37, 40
Thorazine, 34, 35
Tranquilizers, 10, 13
Treatment, 10, 21, 26–44
  early, 9, 14, 78
  in jail, 92, 118
  mandatory outpatient treatment law, 89
  newest, 13, 50, 68–69
  of the homeless, 106–107
  of women, 98–102
Twins, 56–61

V
Violence, 28, 88–92, 106, 116
Vitamins, 36, 38–39
Voices, 4, 16, 90, 95, 115

W
Women's issues, 98–102
  homelessness, 105, 106
World Health Association / Organization.
  See Studies, 23, 47

Z
Zyprexa (olanzapine), 34, 35